COMLEX Level 2-PE
Review Guide

MARK KAUFFMAN, DO, PA
Clinical Associate Professor of Medicine
Director of History and Physical Examination
Lake Erie College of Osteopathic Medicine
Erie, Pennsylvania

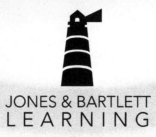

JONES & BARTLETT
LEARNING

World Headquarters
Jones & Bartlett Learning
5 Wall Street
Burlington, MA 01803
978-443-5000
info@jblearning.com
www.jblearning.com

Jones & Bartlett Learning books and products are available through most bookstores and online booksellers. To contact Jones & Bartlett Learning directly, call 800-832-0034, fax 978-443-8000, or visit our website, www.jblearning.com.

Substantial discounts on bulk quantities of Jones & Bartlett Learning publications are available to corporations, professional associations, and other qualified organizations. For details and specific discount information, contact the special sales department at Jones & Bartlett Learning via the above contact information or send an email to specialsales@jblearning.com.

The authors, editor, and publisher have made every effort to provide accurate information. However, they are not responsible for errors, omissions, or for any outcomes related to the use of the contents of this book and take no responsibility for the use of the products and procedures described. Treatments and side effects described in this book may not be applicable to all people; likewise, some people may require a dose or experience a side effect that is not described herein. Drugs and medical devices are discussed that may have limited availability controlled by the Food and Drug Administration (FDA) for use only in a research study or clinical trial. Research, clinical practice, and government regulations often change the accepted standard in this field. When consideration is being given to use of any drug in the clinical setting, the health care provider or reader is responsible for determining FDA status of the drug, reading the package insert, and reviewing prescribing information for the most up-to-date recommendations on dose, precautions, and contraindications, and determining the appropriate usage for the product. This is especially important in the case of drugs that are new or seldom used.

Production Credits
Publisher: David Cella
Associate Editor: Maro Gartside
Editorial Assistant: Teresa Reilly
Production Director: Amy Rose
Associate Production Editor: Julia Waugaman
Marketing Manager: Grace Richards
Manufacturing and Inventory Control Supervisor: Amy Bacus
Composition: Glyph International
Cover Design: Scott Moden
Chapter Opener Image: © Mario Beauregard/ShutterStock, Inc.
Printing and Binding: Edwards Brothers Malloy
Cover Printing: Edwards Brothers Malloy

Library of Congress Cataloging-in-Publication Data
Kauffman, Mark, DO.
  COMLEX level 2-PE review guide/Mark Kauffman.
      p. ; cm.
  Includes bibliographical references and index.
  ISBN 978-0-7637-7654-1 (alk. paper)
  1. Osteopathic medicine—Examinations—Study guides. I. Title.
  [DNLM: 1. Manipulation, Osteopathic—Examination Questions. 2. Clinical
Competence—Examination Questions. 3. Osteopathic Medicine—Examination
Questions. WB 18.2 K21c 2011]
  RZ343.K38 2011
  615.5'33076—dc22
                                                                        2009051176

6048

Printed in the United States of America
17 16 15   10 9 8 7

I would like to dedicate this book to my father, Eugene Kauffman, who once said the job of every father is to make the life of his children better than his own. At this, he has succeeded.

To my wife, Michele, who has brought me three wonderful children, Sam, Kevin, and Jade, and whose patience with me seems eternal.

And to my students, one of whom sat in the front row shaking his head after one lecture. When I asked him what was wrong, he said, "I don't know why you are teaching; you would make such a great practicing physician." With a smile, I replied, "Wouldn't you rather be taught by a good clinical physician who chooses to teach?"

Contents

Introduction   ix
About the Author   xi
Contributors   xiii

Chapter 1

COMLEX Level 2 Performance Examination Overview   1

Eligibility   1
NBOME Website   1
Special Accommodations   1
Testing Site   2
Confidentiality Agreement   2
Structure of the Exam   2
   The Biomedical/Biomechanical Domain   2
   Humanistic Domain   3
Grading   3
Available Resources   4
References   4

Chapter 2

Humanistic Domain   5

Verbal Skills   5
Listening Skills   6
Educational/Instructional Skills   7
Respect   8
Empathy   10
Professionalism   11
References   12

Chapter 3

Biomedical/Biomechanical Domain: Review of Patient Information and Introduction to the Patient   13

Overview of the Standardized
  Patient Encounter   13
The Patient Data Sheet   14
   Patient's Name   14
   Office Setting   14

   Reason for the Visit   15
   Age and Sex   15
   Race   15
   Vital Signs   15
Final Preparation   15
   The Mnemonic: CODIERS SMASH FM   16
Introduction to the Patient   16
Reference   18

Chapter 4

Biomedical/Biomechanical Domain: History Taking   19

History of Present Illness   19
The Opening Statement   19
Open-Ended Questioning   20
Redirection   20
The Chief Complaint   21
Logical Sequence   21
Components of the History of Present Illness:
   CODIERS SMASH FM   22
   CODIERS   22
   SMASH FM   29

Chapter 5

Biomedical/Biomechanical Domain: Physical Examination   35

The Patient Data Sheet   35
Beginning the Examination   36
Comparison of Examination Methods   37
   Case Scenario   37
   Recommended Head-to-Toe Method
     of Examination   37
   The Target Method   40
Prohibited Examinations   41
Tips for Physical Examination by System   41
   Vital Signs   42
   Integumentary Exam   42
   Sensitive Exams: Genital, Breast,
     and Rectal Exams   45
Reference   45

Chapter 6

Biomedical/Biomechanical Domain: Assessment and Plan   47

Assessment   47
  Patients with a Chief Complaint   47
  Patients Without a Chief Complaint   48
  Sharing the Diagnosis with the Patient   49
The Plan   49
  MOTHRR   49
Exiting the Room   53
References   53

Chapter 7

SOAP Note Documentation   55

Theodore Makoske
Writing the SOAP Note   55
Subjective   55
Objective   58
Assessment   59
  Assessment Scoring   60
Plan   60
  MOTHRR   61
False Documentation   62
Stop Writing!   62
SOAP Note Scoring   64
References   64

Chapter 8

Sample Cases   65

Michele M. Roth-Kauffman
What to Expect on the COMLEX 2-PE   65
Anticipated Cases   66
How to Utilize the Practice Cases   66
References   68

Cases

Case 1: An 18 y/o female presents for "a runny nose."   69
Sample SOAP Note Provided for Case 1   73
Case 2: A 45 y/o male presents for "shoulder pain."   75
Sample SOAP Note Provided for Case 2   79
Case 3: A 76 y/o female is brought into your office by her daughter for forgetfulness.   81
Case 4: A 26 y/o female presents c/o foot pain.   85
Case 5: A 62 y/o Caucasian male presents with chest pain.   89
Case 6: A 35 y/o Caucasian male presents with abdominal pain.   93

Case 7: A 35 y/o Caucasian male presents with shortness of breath.   97
Case 8: An 88 y/o male presents with back pain.   101
Case 9: A 15 y/o female presents for "a burn on my forehead."   105
Case 10: A 21 y/o female complaining of a cold.   109
Case 11: An 82 y/o female is brought to the emergency room by ambulance.   113
Case 12: A 24 y/o female presents for "UTI."   117
Case 13: A 72 y/o male presents with leg pain.   121
Case 14: A 25 y/o female presents for "fertility planning."   125
Case 15: A 51 y/o AA male presents for evaluation of blood pressure.   129
Case 16: A 4-month-old male presents with his mother for "spitting up."   133
Case 17: A 30 y/o male presents c/o knee pain.   137
Case 18: A 62 y/o female presents for "coughing all the time."   141
Case 19: A 20 y/o female presents with "My head hurts."   145
Case 20: An 18 y/o female presents with a headache.   149
Case 21: A 49 y/o female presents with neck pain.   153
Case 22: A 68 y/o male presents for "lightheadedness."   157
Case 23: A 57 y/o male presents for shortness of breath.   161
Case 24: A 45 y/o female presents for "swelling of the wrists."   165
Case 25: A 20 y/o female presents for "a rash."   169
Case 26: A 14 y/o female presents for "a hump on her back." Mother is present.   173
Case 27: A 36 y/o female presents for "a cold."   177
Case 28: A 56 y/o female presents c/o lower leg pain.   181
Case 29: A 22 y/o female complaining of no menses for 3 months.   185
Case 30: A 22 y/o male college student presents with chest pain.   189
Case 31: An 82 y/o male presents with a "private problem."   193
Case 32: A 67 y/o Caucasian male presents with a cough.   197

Contents

Case 33: A 43 y/o Caucasian female presents for abdominal pain. 201

Case 34: A 69 y/o male presents for leg pain. 205

Case 35: A 54 y/o female presents with foot pain. 209

Case 36: A 76 y/o male presents with hearing loss. 213

Case 37: A 69 y/o male presents to the office with hematuria. 217

Case 38: A 53 y/o female presents for evaluation of cholesterol. 221

Case 39: A 15 y/o female presents with palpitations. 225

Case 40: A 43 y/o male presents c/o arm pain. 229

Case 41: A 28 y/o Caucasian male presents with back pain. 233

Case 42: A 32 y/o female presents, stating,"I think I'm pregnant." 237

Case 43: A 49 y/o male presents complaining of abdominal pain. 241

Case 44: A 54 y/o female presents c/o arm pain. 245

Case 45: A 42 y/o obese male complains of excessive fatigue. 249

Case 46: A 38 y/o male presents to quit smoking. 253

Case 47: A 79 y/o male presents for "funny heart beats." 257

Case 48: A 62 y/o Vietnamese male presents with a cough (daughter is translating). 261

Case 49: A 32 y/o female presents for "headaches." 265

Case 50: A 68 y/o female presents c/o being up all night going to the bathroom. 269

Appendix A
COMLEX 2-PE Quick Reference Guide **273**

Appendix B
Common Medical Abbreviations **277**

Index **281**

Introduction

The Comprehensive Osteopathic Medical Licensing Examination (COMLEX-USA) is a three-level examination administered by the National Board of Osteopathic Medical Examiners (NBOME) that is designed to document the attainment of national standards in medical knowledge and clinical skills of the candidates of osteopathic medicine.[1p1]

The levels of examination are denoted as COMLEX Level 1, COMLEX Level 2, and COMLEX Level 3, and are formatted as a written examination. In 2004, the addition of the COMLEX Level 2 Performance Evaluation (PE) incorporated the assessment of the osteopathic student's clinical skills to document competency in patient encounters and manipulation that would attest to the safety of delivery of medical care. Level 2 was then designated as having two components: the COMLEX Level 2 Cognitive Evaluation (COMLEX 2-CE) and the COMLEX Level 2-PE.

Levels 2 and 3 of the examination require prior successful passage of the previous COMLEX level. Students must pass both the COMLEX 2-CE and COMLEX 2-PE to be eligible to take the COMLEX Level 3 examination. Successful passage of each level of the COMLEX-USA examination is required for attainment of medical licenses. Currently in development is the fusion of the written examinations into one comprehensive COMLEX exam. The COMLEX 2-PE will continue to be required.

The COMLEX 2-PE format for evaluation consists of standardized patient encounters where candidates interview trained professional patients in mock clinical settings. Patients present a variety of chief complaints that are commonly encountered in primary care settings. These include well visits and acute visits for illness.

For evaluation purposes, the patient encounter is divided into two components. The first component is called the Biomedical/Biomechanical domain and assesses the candidate's ability to take a complete history and perform a physical examination, develop an assessment plan that incorporates osteopathic manipulative medicine (OMM), and document the encounter with a standard subjective, objective, assessment, plan (SOAP) note.[1p17,2]

The second component is the Humanistic domain, an assessment that focuses on the candidate's communication skills during the clinical encounter.

A candidate must pass both domains to pass the examination.

WELL WISHES

Good luck and please feel free to provide both negative and positive feedback, recommendations, and suggestions from your preparation for the COMLEX 2-PE to mkauffman@LECOM.edu. Thank you.

REFERENCES

1. National Board of Osteopathic Medical Examiners. *Bulletin of Information 2009–2010.* Available at: http://nbome.org/docs/comlexBOI.pdf. Accessed November 27, 2008.
2. Gimpel JR, Boulet JR, Errichetti AM. Evaluating the clinical skills of osteopathic medical candidates. *JAOA.* June 2003;103:269-270.

About the Author

Mark Kauffman, DO, PA, is a clinical associate professor of medicine and director of history and physical examination at Lake Erie College of Osteopathic Medicine in Erie, Pennsylvania. He will complete his master's of science degree in Medical Education in April 2010. He was board certified in Family Practice in 2003. His previous text publications include *The History and Physical Examination Workbook: A Common Sense Approach*.

Contributors

Theodore Makoske, MD
Clinical Assistant Professor of Medicine
Clinical Assistant Director of Independent Study
Lake Erie College of Osteopathic Medicine
Erie, Pennsylvania

Michele M. Roth-Kauffman, JD, MPAS, PA-C
Chair, Physician Assistant Department
Gannon University
Erie, Pennsylvania

COMLEX Level 2 Performance Examination Overview

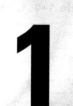
ELIGIBILITY

Eligibility to take the COMLEX-USA Level 2 Performance Examination (COMLEX 2-PE) is determined by several criteria. First, the candidate must be currently enrolled at an osteopathic medical school. The school must be accredited by the American Osteopathic Association's Commission on Osteopathic College Accreditation. The candidate must also have completed the second year of medical school (MS-II) didactic curriculum and passed the COMLEX Level 1 examination. Candidates cannot take the COMLEX Level 2 examination without successful passage of Level 1. In addition, the dean of the candidate's medical school must give approval for the candidate to take the COMLEX 2-PE. There is no required order for taking the COMLEX Level 2 Cognitive Evaluation (COMLEX 2-CE) or the COMLEX 2-PE. Candidates may take either exam first as long as they meet all eligibility criteria. Applicants who have already graduated from an accredited osteopathic medical school can apply by submitting a copy of their diploma.[1p3] Table 1–1 provides a quick reference checklist for COMLEX 2-PE eligibility.

NBOME WEBSITE

Candidates can find all information regarding the COMLEX examination process at the National Board of Osteopathic Medical Examiners (NBOME) web site at www.nbome.org. This is also the route for candidate registration, scheduling, and payment of funds required to take the examination. Candidates cannot schedule their exam until the dean of the candidate's school advises NBOME that the candidate is eligible. Candidates can schedule the COMLEX 2-PE up to 1 year prior to the actual test date. Because available slots fill quickly, candidates should request a test date well in advance. This is especially true if completion of the COMLEX-USA Level 2-PE is required by the candidate's school prior to graduation; in such cases, candidates should schedule the test before January 31 of the year of their predicted graduation.[1p7]

SPECIAL ACCOMMODATIONS

Special accommodations may be available for any candidate with a disability defined by the Americans with Disabilities Act. Candidates must submit applications for accommodations in writing by filling out the correct form, which can be found on the NBOME web site (www.nbome.org).[1p8]

Table 1–1 COMLEX 2-PE Eligibility Checklist

Item	✓
Are you attending an osteopathic medical school?	
Is the medical school accredited by the American Osteopathic Association?	
Have you completed your second year of medical school (MS-II)?	
Have you passed the COMLEX Level 1 Examination?	
Has the dean of your school given approval for you to take the COMLEX Level 2-PE examination?	

TESTING SITE

There is currently only one examination site, the National Center for Clinical Skills Testing, located at 101 West Elm Street, Conshohocken, Pennsylvania, which is in the Philadelphia area. Each candidate must travel to the site to complete the COMLEX 2-PE.[1p16]

CONFIDENTIALITY AGREEMENT

Candidates who take any component of the COMLEX examination are bound by the Candidate Confidentiality Agreement. This agreement, which the candidate must sign, states that all information regarding content of the examination is confidential and cannot be discussed or relayed to any other individual in any manner, including in spoken or printed form. Penalties for violating this agreement can be severe and include the possibility of invalidation and failing of the examination.[1p5]

In this regard, this author made no attempt to obtain content of case samples of the COMLEX 2-PE from prior candidates. However, through literature searches of publications concerning the development of this evaluation tool and publicly available descriptions of the COMLEX 2-PE available from NBOME, this author was able to surmise likely case topics and develop case-based scenarios that likely mimic those that candidates can expect to encounter on the practical examination.

STRUCTURE OF THE EXAM

Candidates complete the COMLEX 2-PE examination in 1 day. Each candidate encounters 12 standardized patients in individual clinical scenarios.[2]

The clinical encounters are timed so that the candidate has 14 minutes to gather the history and perform a problem-specific examination. Then, through problem solving, the candidate must provide the patient with a diagnosis, safely perform osteopathic manipulative medicine (OMM) if appropriate, and develop a treatment plan based on the proposed diagnosis. Following the 14-minute encounter, candidates receive an additional 9 minutes to write a subjective, objective, assessment, plan (SOAP) note documenting the encounter.

The purpose of the examination is to prove the osteopathic medical candidate's competency and ability to safely perform assessment, diagnosis, and treatment using clinical skills. By doing so, licensing bodies have a tool to document public safety.

Clinical skills are defined as patient-centered skills and are evaluated through the candidate's interaction with the standardized patient. Areas evaluated are broken down into two components termed domains: the Biomedical/Biomechanical domain, and the Humanistic domain. These domains are briefly overviewed in the following subsections and discussed in detail in later chapters.

The Biomedical/Biomechanical Domain

The Biomedical/Biomechanical domain concerns medical history taking and physical examination skills, osteopathic manipulative medicine, and the ability to develop a differential diagnosis and associated treatment plan.[2]

The candidate's ability to document the encounter properly is also evaluated. Following the standardized patient encounter, the student immediately documents in the standard SOAP note format

Table 1-2 Components of the Biomedical/Biomechanical Domain

History taking	Obtaining historical data related to the patient's chief complaint
Physical examination	Problem-specific exam dictated by the history
Assessment	Listing differential diagnoses in order of likelihood
Plan	Developing a treatment plan for the proposed diagnoses
Osteopathic manipulation	Educating about and performing osteopathic manipulative medicine if appropriate
Documentation	Recording the encounter through the standard SOAP note

Table 1-3 Components of the Humanistic Domain

Communication skills	Verbal clarity and appropriateness, appropriate nonverbal communication
Interpersonal skills	Demonstration of empathy, helpfulness, and understanding
Professionalism	Dress, demeanor, and clinical competence

the history taken and examination performed including findings, assessment, plans, and manipulation performed. (The SOAP note is discussed in detail in Chapter 7.) A summary of the components of the Biomedical/Biomechanical domain are shown in Table 1-2.

Immediately following each encounter, by completing a checklist the standardized patients evaluate the candidate's history-taking and physical examination skills. The history-taking evaluation assesses whether the candidate asked the appropriate questions based on the patient's chief complaint as well as questions that should have arisen from answers encountered during the patient interview.

The physical examination evaluation contains those parts of the problem-specific examination that the candidate should perform based on the clues obtained in the history. Because time does not allow for comprehensive examinations, this is a focused physical examination based on the chief complaint and likely diagnosis developed during the history taking. Candidates must not only perform the exam, they must perform the exam with technical proficiency.[2]

For example, if a candidate performs auscultation of the lungs but listens only at one level anteriorly or listens through a gown instead of on bare skin, the candidate is not given credit for that part of the examination.

Osteopathic physicians evaluate and grade the candidate's OMM techniques and SOAP note documentation. Osteopathic manipulation is not appropriate for all cases and should not be performed in every scenario.

Humanistic Domain

The standardized patient also completes the Humanistic domain evaluation immediately following the encounter and rates the candidate's competency to communicate in English with the patient and ability to display clarity, professionalism, and empathy.[2] Table 1-3 highlights the components of the Humanistic domain.

GRADING

Percentage grades are derived for each domain of the COMLEX 2-PE. The Biomedical/Biomechanical domain score is composed of adding two thirds of the clinical skills percentage score (incurred through the history taking, physical examination, assessment, plan, and manipulation) with one third of the percentage score obtained from the written SOAP note documentation.[2]

The Humanistic domain score is composed of the standardized patient evaluation of the candidate's communication and relationship skills at each of the 12 patient encounters. Assessment areas include verbal skills, listening skills, instructive skills, respect, empathy, and professionalism. Each area is assigned a grade from 1 to 9 with 9 being the best possible score. The final score for the individual encounter is the mean of each of the preceding six areas.[2]

An overall score is then determined by averaging the 12 case encounters for each domain thereby providing a final score for the Biomedical/Biomechanical and Humanistic domains. This averaging allows the candidate to compensate for substandard performance in one area with consistently superior performance in other areas. For example, if a candidate fails to recognize that manipulation was appropriate for a sinusitis case, the candidate may fail that encounter's Biomedical/Biomechanical domain; however, if the candidate's performance in that domain receives higher grades in other cases, the deficiency is offset.[2]

Grading of the COMLEX 2-PE is pass or fail only. To pass the examination, the candidate must pass both the Biomedical/Biomechanical and Humanistic domains.[1p12]

When a candidate fails the examination, additional information is provided via a grade report that breaks down the scoring in each domain.[3] With this breakdown, the candidate can identify in which domain he or she lacks proficiency. For example, the candidate may be deemed proficient in documenting the history and performing the physical exam, but the candidate may have performed poorly on the osteopathic manipulative treatment (OMT) and SOAP note documentation.

AVAILABLE RESOURCES

The greatest resource available for candidates to familiarize themselves with the policies, procedures, and structure of the COMLEX 2-PE is the NBOME web site (www.nbome.org). Prior to the examination, candidates should take every opportunity to review the *Bulletin of Information*, COMLEX 2-PE Orientation Guide, and the DVD Instructional Program. These highly useful resources provide detailed information on eligibility and examination format. The DVD demonstrates the standardized patient clinical encounter and offers helpful hints such as what equipment is found in the examination rooms. No candidate should miss the opportunity to review this information.

Following is a list of COMLEX 2-PE preparation resources that can be found at the NBOME web site:

- Bulletin of Information
- PE Orientation Guide
- PE Instructional Video

At the NBOME web site, the "For Candidates" tab provides a list of links in the left column. Under the "Testing" link, candidates can click the "COMLEX L2 PE" link to access the preceding resources.

The *Bulletin of Information* is labeled "BOI Document." The "NCCST Info" arrow provides links to the PE Orientation Guide and the PE Instructional Video, which is labeled "Instr Prog DVD."

REFERENCES

1. National Board of Osteopathic Medical Examiners. *Bulletin of Information 2009–2010*. Available at: http://nbome.org/docs/comlexBOI.pdf. Accessed November 27, 2008.
2. Gimpel JR, Boulet JR, Errichetti AM. Evaluating the clinical skills of osteopathic medical candidates. *JAOA*. June 2003;103:268–271.
3. National Board of Osteopathic Medical Examiners. Level 2 Performance Evaluation (PE) FAQ. Available at: http://nbome.org/exams-faqpe.asp. Accessed November 27, 2008.

Humanistic Domain

The COMLEX 2-PE is split into two domains, the Biomedical/Biomechanical domain and the Humanistic domain. Candidates must pass both domains to pass the entire exam successfully. The Humanistic domain focuses on the relationship between the physician and the patient, and in particular, the ability of the physician to communicate properly with the patient. The evaluation of these skills is referred to as the "global patient assessment"[1] and is completed by the standardized patient following the encounter after the candidate has left the examination room. The standardized patient evaluates the following areas: verbal skills, listening skills, educational/instructional skills, respect, empathy, and professionalism.[2p12]

This chapter discusses specific items that relate to each area. A summary table in each section includes proposed standardized patient evaluation.

VERBAL SKILLS

Table 2–1 Verbal Skills: Standardized Patient Checklist

Did the candidate take a thorough history?	Yes	No
Did the candidate speak clearly in English?	Yes	No
Did the candidate speak at an adequate volume level?	Yes	No
Was the candidate's questioning following a logical thought process?	Yes	No
Did the candidate ask appropriate follow-up questions to incomplete answers?	Yes	No
Did the candidate use open-ended questions?	Yes	No
Did the candidate avoid medical jargon?	Yes	No

Content Breakdown:

- Did the candidate ask the appropriate questions leading to a thorough history?
  - **DO:** Utilize the mnemonic CODIERS SMASH FM to obtain a complete history. (See Chapter 4, "Biomedical/Biomechanical Domain: History Taking.")
- Were the questions spoken clearly, in English, with the appropriate level of volume?
  - **DON'T:** Speak with low volumes, mumbling, or heavy accents.
- Were the questions logical?
  - **DON'T:** Jump to another area before completing the current topic.

  Candidate: Did this ever happen before?
  Patient: Yes.

Candidate: Are you on any medications? [Should have asked when it happened before]
Patient: Yes.
Candidate: Do you have a fever? [Should have asked which medications]
Patient: No.

- **DO:** Complete the entire topic area before jumping to another area.

  Candidate: Are you on any medications?
  Patient: Yes.
  Candidate: Which ones?
  Patient: A blood pressure medication.
  Candidate: Do you know the name?
  Patient: Hydrochlorothiazide.
  Candidate: How many milligrams is it?
  Patient: Twenty-five milligrams.
  Candidate: How many times a day do you take it?
  Patient: Just once in the morning.
  Candidate: Are you on any other medications?
  Patient: No.

- Did questions begin with open-ended approaches and move to more specific questioning as needed?
  - **DON'T:** Begin with closed-ended questions.

    Candidate: Is the pain sharp?
    Patient: No.
    Candidate: Is it throbbing?
    Patient: No.

  - **DO:** Begin with open-ended questions and move to closed-ended as needed.

    Candidate: Can you describe the pain? [open-ended]
    Patient: Yes, it hurts.
    Candidate: Can you be more specific? [open-ended]
    Patient: It hurts a lot.
    Candidate: Would you say it is sharp, dull, achy, throbbing . . . ? [closed-ended]
    Patient: It's throbbing.

LISTENING SKILLS

Table 2–2 Listening Skills: Standardized Patient Checklist

Did the candidate recognize and respond to historical clues?	Yes	No
Did the candidate repeat questions that were already answered?	Yes	No
Did the candidate legitimize your concerns?	Yes	No

Content Breakdown:

- Did the candidate react to historical clues by asking appropriate follow-up questions?
  - **DON'T:** Ignore historical prompts.

    Candidate: Did anything make it worse?
    Patient: Standing too long on it.
    Candidate: Did anything make it better? [Should have asked what the patient does that requires him or her to stand for long periods]
    Patient: Not really.

  - **DO:** Follow historical leads.

    Candidate: Did this ever happen before?
    Patient: Yes.
    Candidate: When was that?
    Patient: About 2 months ago.

Candidate: How was it treated?
Patient: They gave me ibuprofen.
Candidate: Did that help?
Patient: Yes. It was gone in 2 days.
Candidate: What was the diagnosis?
Patient: They said it was a mild sprain.

- Did the candidate ask the same questions over again?
  - **DON'T:** Ask the same questions over again.

    Candidate: How did this happen?
    Patient: I was bit by a dog while delivering the mail.
    Candidate: When was that?
    Patient: Two days ago.
    Candidate: Did you see anyone for it then?
    Patient: No.

    Followed later by:

    Candidate: What do you do for a living?
    Patient: I deliver mail. [already stated by patient]
- Did the candidate acknowledge concerns expressed by the patient?
  - **DON'T:** Skip clues about patient concerns.

    Patient: That medicine must be expensive.
    Candidate: Yes, medicine can be costly.
  - **DO:** Acknowledge patient concerns.

    Patient: That medicine must be expensive.
    Candidate: Do you have insurance?
    Patient: No.
    Candidate: Let's think about less expensive alternatives then.

EDUCATIONAL/INSTRUCTIONAL SKILLS

Table 2–3 Educational/Instructional Skills: Standardized Patient Checklist

Did the candidate provide you with a diagnosis?	Yes	No
Was the diagnosis clearly explained?	Yes	No
Did the candidate include you in the development of a treatment plan?	Yes	No
Were you provided with a treatment plan?	Yes	No
Was the treatment plan logical?	Yes	No
Was the treatment plan easily understood?	Yes	No
Did the candidate address your concerns?	Yes	No
Did the candidate ask if you had any questions?	Yes	No
Did the candidate thank you at the end of the encounter?	Yes	No

Content Breakdown:

- Did the candidate provide a diagnosis?
  Candidates must always present the patient with a proposed diagnosis, even if they are not sure of what the diagnosis is. For example, a patient presents with chest pain that occurs with deep respiration. The candidate elicits both musculoskeletal and respiratory components through the history taking and physical examination. In the differential, the candidate suspects a rib dysfunction as the most likely diagnosis, but also considers pneumonia to be a weaker possibility.

  Candidate: Mrs. Kendziora, I think this pain is coming from a dysfunction of your rib cage; however, there is a chance you have pneumonia, so I'll also be sending you for chest X-ray.

Here, the candidate proposes a diagnosis, and the plan includes ruling out other diagnoses in the differential.

- Did the candidate clearly explain the diagnosis?

    Candidate: Mrs. Kendziora, when we breathe, our ribs need to move freely. Sometimes our ribs get stuck in the wrong position, which can cause us to have chest pain. I think this is what is causing your pain.

    This explanation is short, simple, and to the point and uses terminology the patient can understand.

- Did the candidate provide a plan of treatment?

    Candidate: Mrs. Kendziora, we've used manipulation on you in the past. This is another time when manipulation can help. With your permission I would like to try it again. I would also like you to take a medication that will help with pain and inflammation.

- Was the treatment plan easy to understand and logical? Following the manipulation:

    Candidate: I did find some dysfunction of your ribs. The manipulation will help, but I'd also like you to take 400 mg of ibuprofen, 3 times a day, with food for the next 2 days. You take it with food to protect your stomach. There is a chance that you have an early pneumonia, so I'd like you to go for an X-ray of your chest right after leaving here. The results will come back to me tomorrow, and I will call you to see how you're feeling and to go over the results with you. I'm not going to start an antibiotic unless the X-ray shows that it's necessary. How does that sound?

- Did the candidate involve the patient in treatment decision making?

    A patient needs a medication for high cholesterol, but has not tried dieting and exercise. The candidate should ask the patient which route he would like to take.

    Candidate: Mr. Feldman, diet and exercise are recommended as first-line treatments for high cholesterol. Do you think you can successfully start avoiding fats and begin an exercise program, or would you rather start the medication?

    Here, the candidate involved the patient in the treatment plan. When physicians involve patients in their own treatment plan, patients are more likely to follow the plan because they now "own" it.

- Did the candidate address the patient's concerns?

    Candidate: Mrs. Kendziora, I want you to go straight to the hospital and get an X-ray taken.

    Patient: But, Doctor, my husband has the car and won't be home until 6 pm.

    Candidate: Oh, I didn't mean to make you feel this was an emergency. The radiology department is open until 10 pm. Can you go after he gets home?

    Patient: Oh, sure.

- Did the candidate offer to include family members in the patient's management?

    Patient: So, Doctor, this type of skin cancer isn't the one that kills people?

    Candidate: This is a basal cell carcinoma, which very rarely goes elsewhere in the body and is usually cured by having it taken completely off.

    Patient: When I tell my wife I have cancer, she is going to be so upset.

    Candidate: Why don't you bring her in so that I can explain it to her? We just have to make sure we keep an eye on the area after we remove the affected tissue to make sure it doesn't come back. I think she'll feel better if we tell her how closely we're going to watch you afterward.

RESPECT

Content Breakdown:

Respect, by definition, means (1) to hold in esteem or honor, and (2) to show regard or consideration for.[3] Part of the humanistic evaluation performed by the standardized patient centers around respect shown during the encounter. As mentioned previously, candidates should regard standardized patient encounters as real patient visits. A candidate with the mind-set that it doesn't really matter that the diagnosis or plan isn't perfect because it won't in reality actually affect the standardized patient will have a very difficult time demonstrating true respect for the patient. Respect for patients must be genuine.

Table 2–4 Respect: Standardized Patient Checklist

Was the candidate polite?	Yes	No
Did the candidate introduce himself/herself?	Yes	No
Did the candidate ask how you would like to be addressed?	Yes	No
Did the candidate shake your hand?	Yes	No
Did the candidate wash his/her hands before touching you?	Yes	No
Did the candidate rewash his/her hands if he/she contaminated himself/herself?	Yes	No
Did you feel the candidate understood your concerns?	Yes	No
Did the candidate demonstrate kindness by helping you with position changes?	Yes	No
Did the candidate appropriately drape you to preserve dignity when exposing you for examination?	Yes	No
Did the candidate ask permission before exposing any body area?	Yes	No
Did the candidate respect your right to choose as a patient?	Yes	No
Did you feel cultural differences were respected?	Yes	No
Did you feel that you were held in high esteem?	Yes	No

It is easy to become cynical in the practice of medicine, yet the best physician is one who leaves prejudice at the door when walking into a room. Minimally, candidates must adopt the mind-set that the standardized patient has invested in them as physicians in training and is helping candidates to become good physicians. Candidates must be appreciative of the role standardized patients play. Ultimately, they must see the patient as someone in their office with whom they are forging a relationship and for whom they will provide a lifetime of care.

- Was the candidate polite?
  - ➢ Candidates should introduce themselves using their name and title.
  - ➢ They should use the patient's full name.
  - ➢ They should ask what the patient would prefer to be called.
  - ➢ They should thank the patient at the end of the session.

- Did the candidate show sensitivity?
  - ➢ Candidates should demonstrate understanding of the concern the patient has.
  - ➢ They should demonstrate kindness by helping the patient make position changes.
  - ➢ They should demonstrate warmth by shaking the patient's hand.
  - ➢ Candidates must properly drape the patient's lower extremities when performing an abdominal examination to avoid exposure of the pelvic region when lifting up the gown. Ask permission to do so.

- Did the candidate respect the patient's right to choose?
  - ➢ A candidate offers smoking cessation to a patient. The candidate should explore what attempts the patient made in the past and how well these worked. The candidate can ask the patient what she thinks will work best to help her quit successfully.

- Did the candidate respect cultural differences and backgrounds?
  - ➢ A Middle Eastern couple comes into the clinic. The husband explains that his wife has a cough. The candidate is a male physician and recognizes that he needs the husband's permission to examine his wife. The husband will not allow it. The candidate does not get angry, stating that he can't treat the woman without listening to her chest, but instead finds an alternative, such as asking his female office partner to perform the examination.

- Did the patient feel that he was respected and held in high esteem?
  - ➢ Candidates can demonstrate that they appreciate the patient's being there by thanking them.

EMPATHY

Content Breakdown:

Synonyms for *empathy* include understanding, sympathy, and compassion. Empathy can be expressed both verbally and nonverbally. Eye contact is important in developing a bond with the patient. The expression "the eyes are the windows to the soul" reflects on humans' ability to communicate with their eyes alone. Patients typically like eye contact about 50% of the time, but the amount used should be based on the individual encounter. Elderly patients may desire more, younger patients less. By making eye contact initially on entering a room, physicians can forge an early bond with patients. On the other hand, when physicians walk in while staring at their papers and charts, they may appear distant and mechanical and lacking in compassion.

- Did the candidate demonstrate compassion and sympathy?
  - ➤ Mr. Jones had his gallbladder removed last year. Since that time, fatty foods have caused him to have episodes of urgent diarrhea. Twice he has been eating out and barely made it to the restroom in time. The candidate should discuss with him how this situation is limiting his lifestyle.

- Did the candidate show interest in the patient's condition?
  - ➤ Telling the patient, "It's just a cold virus. You'll get better" shows the patient very little investment. The patient has invested a great deal to come to see the physician: she has scheduled an appointment, taken a day off work, waited in a crowded waiting room with sick people all around, remained calm when the physician was running an hour late, and waited in the exam room for another half hour. Although the diagnosis that the patient just has a virus that will run its course in a few days may be correct, there are better ways to tell the patient and show interest in his or her condition. Obviously, the condition is a concern for the patient. Candidates must decide which symptoms they can treat. Does the patient need a decongestant or cough suppressant? Would manipulation benefit the patient? Does she need a day or two off from work so that the virus isn't spread?

- Did the candidate acknowledge the patient's life situation?
  - ➤ Eugene injured his rotator cuff. This condition is aggravated by his occupation as a roofer. The candidate advises Eugene that he needs to take a week off from his work to allow his shoulder to begin healing.

    Patient: A week off? Doc, roofing doesn't happen in the wintertime. If don't work, I don't get paid. We don't have sick time.

    Candidate: I see. This will definitely make healing much more of a challenge, but let's think this through and figure out the best way to help you.

- Did the candidate acknowledge and demonstrate understanding of how the current condition would affect the patient's life?

  Candidates must consider how patients' current conditions will affect their ability to work or participate in activities of daily living.
  - ➤ Mrs. Wagaman is 93 years old and just fractured her right wrist. The candidate must consider whether she lives alone. Can she drive back home and take care of herself once she gets there? The candidate should ask the patient if there is anyone he can call to discuss her condition and needs with. She has three children in town; could she live with anyone while she recovers?

Table 2–5 Empathy: Standardized Patient Checklist

Did the candidate demonstrate compassion and sympathy?	Yes	No
Did the candidate show interest in your condition and recognize its importance to you?	Yes	No
Did the candidate acknowledge your current life situation?	Yes	No
Did the candidate understand the affect your current condition would have on your work, home, or activities?	Yes	No
Did the candidate make appropriate eye contact?	Yes	No

PROFESSIONALISM

Content Breakdown:

Professionalism is judged not only by how candidates act, but also by how they appear. Although professionalism goes beyond simple appearance, physical appearance is the first thing the patient sees when the physician enters the room. Patient impressions of competency of care directly relate to their physician's physical appearance: the better dressed the physician, the better the quality of care the patient perceives. Candidates should pay as close attention to their physical appearance as they did when they interviewed for medical school. Their white coat should be clean and wrinkle free. Hygiene is important as well and sometimes it is easy to overlook any deficiencies in this area. Candidates should shower the evening before or the morning of the examination. Their hair should be well groomed, and men who do not have beards should be clean shaven. Beards should be well trimmed and groomed. Clothing should be professional attire: women's clothing should not be too revealing, jewelry should be modest, and men should avoid jewelry and wear a tie.

- Was the candidate dressed professionally and well groomed?
  - ➤ Was the candidate's white coat clean and pressed, or were the cuffs dirt stained?
  - ➤ Did the candidate's shirt reveal cleavage?
  - ➤ Was the candidate wearing a tie?
  - ➤ Did the candidate have a five o'clock shadow?
  - ➤ Was the candidate's makeup too heavy?
  - ➤ Did the candidate wear too much perfume or cologne?
  - ➤ Did the candidate have body odor?
  - ➤ Was the candidate's shirt tucked in?
  - ➤ Was the candidate's hair combed and brushed?
  - ➤ Did the candidate have bad breath?
  - ➤ Did the candidate smell like alcohol?

  Although these guidelines seem too obvious and like they are just common sense, it is worthwhile for candidates to pay close attention to them.

- Did the candidate demonstrate humane concern for the patient? That is, was the candidate kind to the patient?
  - ➤ Candidates must identify with the patient's condition. If a patient presents in pain, the candidate must recognize it and discuss it directly so that the patient understands the pain is a priority for the candidate as well.

    Candidate: Ms. Green, I can see that you are in a lot of pain. I'll help you as quickly as I can.

- Was the candidate confident?
  - ➤ Candidates must avoid "um" and awkward periods of silence. On the patient information sheet, they can write down the mnemonic for history taking: CODIERS SMASH FM. (See also Chapter 4, "Biomedical/Biomechanical Domain: History Taking.") If they get stuck, they can fall back on this.

Table 2–6 Professionalism: Standardized Patient Checklist

Was the candidate professionally dressed and groomed?	Yes	No
Did the candidate have anything in his/her mouth during the encounter?	Yes	No
Did the candidate demonstrate compassion? Was the candidate kind?	Yes	No
Did the candidate appear confident?	Yes	No
Did you feel as if your conversation with the candidate would be kept confidential?	Yes	No
Did the candidate appear ethical?	Yes	No

> After candidates perform the examination, even if they are not completely sure of the diagnosis, they must dedicate themselves to the most likely diagnosis and develop a treatment plan. They can write the plan mnemonic MOTHRR on their patient information sheet, and work through it concisely, advising the patient of each component as they go. (See Chapter 6, "Biomedical/Biomechanical Domain: Assessment and Plan.")

> **Candidate:** Mr. Clark, it looks like you have appendicitis. We'll be moving rather quickly. We need to draw some blood and I'll send you over for a CT scan. I've paged Dr. Gemma to come take a look at you because you might need to go to surgery. The nurse will be putting an IV in so that we can give you an antibiotic and fluids. Unfortunately, you can't have anything to eat or drink. As soon as Dr. Gemma sees you, I'll give you something for your pain. He's on his way. Do you have any questions?

- Did the patient feel as if the information shared would be kept confidential?
  > At times, it is important to assure patients directly that any information they share with the physician will be kept confidential. These times often center around sensitive issues such as sexuality, infectious disease, and mental health, among others. Candidates should ask patients if there is anyone that they would like the candidate to talk to about the patient's condition. This tells patients that unless they give the physician permission, the physician will not share the information with anyone.

  > **Candidate:** Mary, I think the abdominal pain and sleeplessness you're experiencing are symptoms of depression. We can work on this together. Is there anyone you would like me to share this information with?

- Did the candidate appear ethical?
  > Ethics in medicine speaks to principled, just treatment and interactions with patients. Relationships must be on professional levels. For example, overly friendly gestures, such as touching a patient on the leg, could be considered flirtatious and inappropriate. Though encounters with standardized patients will likely leave little room for unethical behavior, it should be guarded against. How would an ethical practitioner respond to this question?

  > **Patient:** Dr. Shen, I know my leg doesn't look too bad, but this week is deer season and I haven't got my buck yet. Do you think I could have a few more days off from work?

A combined summary of the Humanistic domain standardized patient evaluation appears in Appendix A, "COMLEX 2-PE Quick Reference Guide."

REFERENCES

1. Gimpel JR, Boulet JR, Errichetti AM. Evaluating the clinical skills of osteopathic medical candidates. *JAOA*. June 2003;103:269–271.
2. National Board of Osteopathic Medical Examiners. *Bulletin of Information 2009–2010*. Available at: http://nbome.org/docs/comlexBOI.pdf. Accessed November 27, 2008.
3. Dictionary.com. Respect. Available at: http://dictionary.reference.com/browse/respect. Accessed December 6, 2008.

Biomedical/Biomechanical Domain: Review of Patient Information and Introduction to the Patient

As outlined earlier, the Biomedical/Biomechanical domain focuses on three major components:

- *Data gathering:* Obtaining a history and performing a physical examination
- *Osteopathic manipulative treatment (OMT):* Patient education and performance
- *Documentation:* Recording the encounter in standard subjective, objective, assessment, plan (SOAP) note format

This chapter discusses the importance of reviewing patient information prior to entering the patient's room and techniques that candidates can use to introduce themselves when they first enter the room, the first steps in data gathering.

OVERVIEW OF THE STANDARDIZED PATIENT ENCOUNTER

The COMLEX 2-PE test center is designed to replicate a standard outpatient primary care office setting. Each examination room is equipped to meet the demands of a typical outpatient visit. The only personal examination equipment the candidate is required to bring is a stethoscope.[1p3]

On the scheduled day of the COMLEX 2-PE, the candidate encounters 12 different standardized patients. The case format for each patient encounter is the same: the candidate is given 14 minutes to complete the entire encounter, followed by 9 minutes to complete documentation of the encounter in SOAP note format.[1pp4,6]

At the beginning of each case, the candidate can approach the assigned room. An overhead announcement advises the student when the 14-minute patient encounter begins. At that time, the student can open the pull-down wall unit to access a patient data sheet or "doorway information sheet"[1p6] that contains introductory information about the patient. This represents a typical previsit screening and includes the patient's name, visit location, chief complaint, and vital signs. After reviewing this information, the student enters the room and takes a history based on the chief complaint and performs a problem-specific examination.

Another overhead prompt alerts the student when 2 minutes are remaining in the encounter. At this point, the candidate should wrap up the current examination and proceed with assessment and plan, discussing a diagnosis with the patient and developing a plan of therapy. Candidates should ask the patient if he or she has any questions and express gratitude by thanking the patient. When the announcement is made that encounter time is ended, the student must immediately leave the room.

When the start of the SOAP note documentation session is announced, candidates have 9 minutes to complete the SOAP note. Another 2-minute warning is made as the session nears its end. After 9 minutes, the close of the documentation session is announced and the candidate must immediately stop writing. Failure to do so may result in invalidation of that documentation session.

If candidates complete the patient encounter before the 14 minutes is over, they may leave the exam room and begin the SOAP note immediately, thus gaining extra time for documentation. For example, if the candidate completes her patient encounter and leaves the exam room with 4 minutes of the 14-minute session remaining, she can begin the SOAP note and have a total of 13 minutes for documentation—4 left over from the encounter and 9 from the allotted SOAP note documentation time. Candidates must beware that once they leave the exam room, they cannot reenter the room under any circumstances. Therefore, candidates might find that it is better to use any extra time in the patient encounter to further develop a patient–provider relationship.

THE PATIENT DATA SHEET

Prior to entering the room, the candidate should take a short time to become familiar with the information found on the patient data sheet. Each patient information sheet may contain the following information:

- Patient name
- Office setting
- Reason for the visit
- Age
- Sex
- Race
- Screening vital signs

Examples can be found at the beginning of each case in Chapter 8 and on the NBOME web site (www.nbome.org) on page 6 of the *2008–2009 Orientation Guide* for the COMLEX-USA Level 2-PE.

Other information may be found with the patient data sheet such as parental consent if the patient is a minor, laboratory values, radiographic images, or electrocardiographs (ECGs).[1p5]

Patient's Name

A proper introduction when entering the patient room sets the foundation for developing good physician–patient rapport. Walking in the room and saying, "Hello, Ms . . . umm . . . Smith," while clumsily looking for her name on the chart, simply tells the patient that the physician is too busy to take a moment to recognize her as a person and not just the next problem on the schedule. Conversely, after candidates review the patient's name and information outside the room, by walking in saying, "Hello, Mrs. Smith, I'm Student Doctor Adams. It's a pleasure to meet you. Would you prefer I call you Mrs. Smith or Linda?" they tell the patient that despite the fact that they have not met each other before, the physician already knows the patient by name and as a person with preferences and valuable opinions.

Office Setting

The candidate should identify the type of facility where the encounter occurs. Based on information provided about typical patient chief complaints, the types of facilities expected would be ambulatory primary care clinics, outpatient offices, or emergency rooms.[1p4]

The location makes a difference particularly when designing a treatment plan for the proposed diagnosis. For example, if the office setting is a family practice clinic and upon entering the room and performing the exam, the candidate determines that the patient may have acute coronary syndrome, his primary concern would be emergent transfer of the patient. The candidate should explain this need to the patient. The SOAP note plan would demonstrate that the candidate is following Advanced Cardiac Life Support (ACLS) guidelines, which include administering aspirin, nitroglycerine, and oxygen while awaiting arrival of the ambulance. The candidate would also notify the hospital of the pending transfer and any family members the patient would like to be notified.

However, if the office setting were the emergency room, the plan would concentrate on diagnostic and treatment protocols. The candidate would advise the patient of the need for admission and referral to the cardiovascular service, with the possibility of the need for cardiac catheterization depending on the results of the evaluation. The SOAP note would document a plan that would administer the patient aspirin, nitroglycerine, and oxygen; however, the candidate would go further in considering a beta-blocker and morphine. Of course, the candidate would place the patient on a monitor, perform serial ECGs, take a chest radiograph, and order stat lab work such as a CBC, chemistry, coagulation, and cardiac profiles.

Reason for the Visit

Often documented by ancillary medical staff, the patient information sheet will contain the reason the patient is there to see you. In clinical practice, the reason for their visit that patients give the nurse might not be the same reason they tell the physician. In these cases, the reason for the visit told to the nurse is called an "admission ticket" and may be offered in cases of embarrassment or concerning other sensitive issues. Therefore, it is important that candidates do not enter the patient room and say something like, "I see you're here for abdominal pain" because the patient may lose courage about admitting the real reason for the visit is depression. Instead, a physician's opening question should allow the patient to tell why he or she is there, such as, "What brings you in today?"

That said, candidates should not expect the reason for the visit as documented on the patient information sheet during the COMLEX 2-PE to be inaccurate. Once confirmed, the reason for the visit is documented as the chief complaint in the Subjective (S) part of the SOAP note.

Age and Sex

Within the patient demographics, age and sex can allow for ranking of the possible diagnoses by likelihood. Using the previous chest pain example, if a 65-year-old man presents with substernal chest pain, the candidate would rank acute coronary syndrome high on the list of possible diagnoses. This diagnosis would be less likely if the patient were a 12-year-old girl—although it is possible that she is having a myocardial infarction, it is highly unlikely.

Race

Race plays a role in the development of a differential diagnosis based on epidemiology of disease. For example, sickle cell disease is much more common in patients of African descent and must be considered with greater suspect in a 12-year-old African American boy with acute left upper quadrant pain than it is in a 12-year-old boy of European descent.

Race may also come into play during treatment planning. For example, when treating a hypertensive African American patient, a physician might choose a calcium channel blocker over a beta-blocker because this population is more responsive to the former.

Vital Signs

Vital signs often include height, weight, temperature, pulse rate, blood pressure, and respiratory rate. Again, these values are typically obtained by ancillary staff before the patient sees the physician. In the COMLEX 2-PE, the accuracy of the previsit screening vitals should not be questioned. There is no need to reobtain the patient's height, weight, or temperature. It would, however, be prudent for candidates to repeat blood pressure, pulse, or respiratory rates when any of these values are abnormal.

For example, if the previsit screen documents a blood pressure of 160/92 mm HG and the candidate repeats the blood pressure in both arms and obtains a 128/70 mm HG right and 124/68 mm HG left, the candidate would not ignore the original elevated measurement, but should include it and plan for appropriate follow-up, perhaps another measurement in a week or so.

On the patient information sheet, candidates may consider circling abnormal vital signs to prompt themselves to repeat these measures as they finish history taking and move on to the physical examination.

FINAL PREPARATION

Candidates have gone to their assigned rooms. An overhead announcement tells them that they may enter the room. This is the beginning of the 14-minute patient encounter. Before going into the room, candidates must open the wall unit and remove the information inside. They must look at the patient

Table 3-1 Patient Data Sheet Example

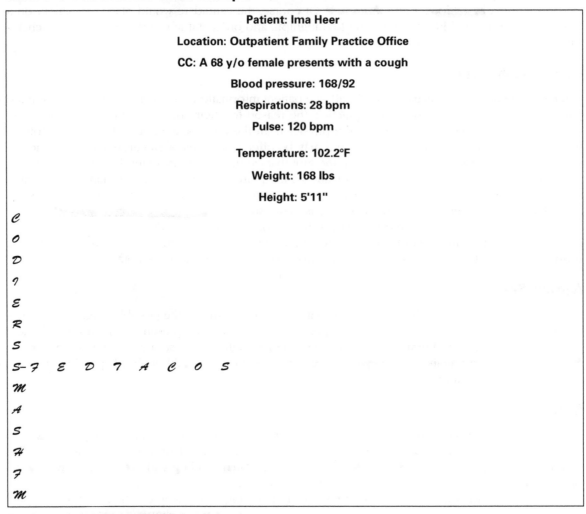

Patient: Ima Heer

Location: Outpatient Family Practice Office

CC: A 68 y/o female presents with a cough

Blood pressure: 168/92

Respirations: 28 bpm

Pulse: 120 bpm

Temperature: 102.2°F

Weight: 168 lbs

Height: 5'11"

C
O
D
I
E
R
S
S-F   E   D   I   A   C   O   S
M
A
S
H
F
M

data and note the location of the visit; the reason the patient gave for the appointment; the age, sex, and race of the patient; and scan the vital signs, circling any abnormalities. In all, this takes about 15 to 30 seconds.

The Mnemonic: CODIERS SMASH FM

Before opening the door, candidates can give themselves something to fall back on. They can write down along the left side of their paper this mnemonic: CODIERS SMASH FM. It is the key to a comprehensive, detailed, yet speedy history. See Table 3–1. The full meaning of the mnemonic is discussed in detail in Chapter 4, "Biomedical/Biomechanical Domain: History Taking."

INTRODUCTION TO THE PATIENT

Introduction of the candidate to the patient involves entering the patient's room, introducing themselves, washing their hands, and the beginning of candidate-patient bonding.

When the candidate enters the room, she must have the mind-set that this is a real patient that she is about to see and must treat him or her as such. If candidates enter the room thinking that this is just a test with a programmed standardized patient who has the answers to all of the questions, they become mechanical, simply try to ask enough questions to pass the exam, and will fail in the Humanistic domain. (See Chapter 2.)

The first few seconds of the patient encounter are crucial for developing a physician–patient relationship. Almost immediately, physicians can run into a problem. It is typical in the United States to greet most patients with a handshake. Unfortunately, if the physician does so prior to washing his or her hands, the physician has just contaminated the patient. Although the candidate might have just washed her hands upon leaving the last room, she had to turn the door handle on the door to get into this room, so whatever is on that handle is now on her hands.

Although it may seem awkward, candidates should knock, enter the room, stop, make eye contact with the patient, greet the patient using his or her name, and introduce themselves. Then, they can briefly excuse themselves to wash their hands in the sink in the examination room while explaining the need to do this before touching the patient. The dialogue may go something like this:

> **Candidate:** Hello, Mr. Roth. I'm Student Doctor Adams. I'll be seeing you today. Please excuse me a few seconds while I wash my hands. I wouldn't want to pass anything along to you.

The patient will be more than happy to postpone the handshake until the candidate washes her hands.

The hand washing period represents the next opportunity for developing the physician–patient relationship. A proper hand washing lasts at least 15 seconds. (See Table 3–2.) Although it sounds basic, the standardized patients are trained to observe for proper hand washing technique as well as to document recontamination of candidates' hands after they have washed. If candidates recontaminate themselves such as by turning off the water with their hand, dropping a pencil on the floor and picking it up, touching their hair or face, or sneezing into their hands, they must rewash.

Before getting down to the business of taking a history of the patient, the 15 seconds of hand washing can begin building a relationship. Instead of jumping in with, "What brings you in today?" candidates can use this time to show the patient that they care for him or her as more than just a symptom. While candidates wash their hands, they might have the following conversation:

> **Candidate:** Mr. Roth, do you prefer to be called Mr. Roth or John?
> **Patient:** Actually, you can call me "Jack."
> **Candidate:** That would be fine, Jack. Did you make it in okay today?
> **Patient:** Yes, no problem at all.
> **Candidate:** Great. I know Philadelphia can get slippery this time of year.
> **Patient:** Oh, I've lived here all of my life. I'm used to it.

The patient perceives that the physician has time for and interest in him or her beyond the sterility of an office visit. By asking the patient's name preference, candidates immediately tell the patient that he has choices to make during the visit, that they will not be dictating everything that occurs, and

Table 3–2 Proper Hand Washing Technique

Ensure paper towel will be able to be retrieved without touching the wall unit.
Turn on hot and cold water and adjust to warm.
Take soap from the dispenser.
Lather for 15 seconds. (This is about the amount of time it takes to sing the ABCs or the Happy Birthday song.)
Rinse your hands.
Take several paper towels to dry your hands, leaving the water running.
Throw the towels away.
Take a fresh paper towel and turn off the water. Do not use this same paper towel to dry your hands further after turning off the water as this is a recontamination.

that his opinion matters. After candidates finish washing their hands, they can walk back over to the patient. So far, the candidate has been in the room for about half a minute and now it's time for business. Candidates should shake the patient's hand and say something like:

> **Candidate:** Jack. It's really nice to meet you. What brings you in today?

REFERENCE

1. National Board of Osteopathic Medical Examiners. *2009–2010 Orientation Guide COMLEX-USA Level 2-PE*. Available at: http://nbome.org/docs/PEOrientationGuide.pdf. Accessed October 9, 2009.

Biomedical/Biomechanical Domain: History Taking

The candidate's competency in data collection in the Biomedical/Biomechanical domain begins with an evaluation of the candidate's ability to take a thorough history.

HISTORY OF PRESENT ILLNESS

The history of present illness (HPI) is the subjective story the patient gives to the candidate in response to questions the candidate poses. Candidates document answers in the Subjective part of the subjective, objective, assessment, plan (SOAP) note, as discussed in Chapter 7, "SOAP Note Documentation." Candidates can think of the *subjective* in the SOAP note as *subject* to change.

THE OPENING STATEMENT

Each history begins with the reason for the patient visit. One of the keys to obtaining an accurate history is to allow the patient to tell his or her story first. As discussed previously, using an open-ended question, candidates should ask patients why they are there to see a physician so that patients can start to tell their story. *Open-ended* simply means that the question cannot be answered with a "yes" or "no" response; such questions require further explanation. Candidates can use any open-ended opening statement they wish as long as it prompts patients to start their story. Good open-ended opening statements are like these:

- "What brings you in today?"
- "How can I help you?"
- "What seems to be the concern today?"

Candidates should avoid an opening statement that may be considered rude or offensive, despite their intentions, such as:

Candidate: What's your problem today?

Also, candidates must avoid restating the reason for the patient visit as documented on the patient data sheet because the patient may state one reason for the visit to the nurse during screening, yet tell a different reason to the physician. For example, Jim, a 75-year-old man, may be embarrassed to tell the 20-year-old nurse that he has difficulty maintaining an erection, so he says he has a problem with his cholesterol pill instead. The nurse documents "Problem with cholesterol pill" as the reason for the patient visit. As the physician enters, he says:

Physician: Jim, it's nice to see you again. I see you have a concern with your cholesterol pill. What's going on?

Jim, who is now embarrassed for misleading the nurse, spends the next 10 minutes discussing the mild fatigue he has after taking his pill. The physician performs an exam and discusses alternatives to Jim's current medication. As the physician is about to leave the room, Jim says:

Patient: One more thing, Doc. . . . You know, I've been having a hard time keeping an erection.

This was the true reason the patient was here to see the physician, and now the visit has to start all over again. This could have been avoided if the physician's opening statement had been more open ended:

Physician: Jim, nice to see you again. What brings you in today?
Patient: Hi, Doc, nice to see you too. It's a bit embarrassing, but I'm here because I'm having a difficult time keeping an erection.
Physician: I see the nurse noted you were having a problem with your cholesterol pill.
Patient: Well, I thought that might be contributing to the problem, but honestly, this has been going on longer than I have been on that pill.

OPEN-ENDED QUESTIONING

The use of open-ended questioning allows patients to use their own words instead of words healthcare providers put into their mouths. If a response fails to provide enough details, candidates can follow the original open-ended question with another open-ended question or statement.

Patient: I have chest pain.
Candidate: Oh, tell me more about that. [open-ended question]

If a patient is unable to answer an open-ended question, candidates may then move on to closed-ended questions, or those that require a yes or no answer or a more specific response. For example:

Candidate: Can you describe the chest pain? [open-ended]
Patient: I don't know. It just hurts. [vague response]
Candidate: Is it is sharp, dull, achy, pressure, squeezing, burning . . . ? [closed-ended]

The patient will typically pick the closest description of the pain when the candidate names it.

REDIRECTION

Candidates must be careful not stray too far away from the main course of questioning or to follow one path into too much detail because the 14-minute time limitation does not allow for it. For example, if a 35-year-old male patient presents with a possible ligamental injury to the knee incurred while playing basketball, obtaining a detailed family history in unnecessary because this information does not contribute to the case.

Candidates might also need to redirect patients if their story begins to diverge too far from the primary concern:

Patient: Well, the first time I had chest pain was back in 1962, when I was visiting my sister Gwendolyn in Florida. Lovely place she has really. Her house was built back in the 1920s. Once she found an original painting by . . .

If the candidate does not redirect this patient, he would need to have pizza sent in for dinner! A candidate's response to this type of stream of consciousness can be something like the following:

Candidate: I'm sorry to interrupt, and if we have time, we can come back to that, but can you tell me when you had the chest pain last?

It may take several redirections in a case like this to keep the patient's information on track. Notice that this second question is more specific than the first.

THE CHIEF COMPLAINT

The reason patients give for their visit is the chief complaint (CC) in the documentation and is a start to their story. For example,

> **Candidate:** Jack. What brings you in today?
> **Patient:** I think I have pneumonia.

Or

> **Patient:** Just getting my diabetes checked.

Or

> **Patient:** I have a ringing in my ears.

Typically, the reason the patient gives the candidate is the same one that the patient provided during the previsit screen, but occasionally these reasons may be different, as discussed earlier.

Sometimes, patients offer a diagnosis such as Jack did with "I think I have pneumonia." The patient may in fact be correct in the diagnosis because, often, no one knows the patient better than himself or herself. However, other conditions may have similar symptoms, and candidates must consider them. If the patient offers a diagnosis, candidates can add it to their differential diagnoses but must keep the differential open to other possibilities.

The chief complaint may also include duration of time. For example:

- CC: "I have chest pain" × 3 hours.
- CC: "I have chest pain" × 23 years.

By using duration of time, the candidate can rank diagnoses in the differential in order of likelihood. The sense of urgency for the patient reporting 3 hours of chest pain varies greatly from the patient with 23 years of chest pain. Of course, there is an overlapping of possibilities, but urgency of evaluation is somewhat diminished in the patient with 23 years of chest pain as compared to that of the patient with 3 hours of pain.

During patient encounters in clinical practice, patients typically answer many questions before physicians can even ask. For example:

> **Physician:** Jack, what brings you in today?
> **Patient:** I have this chest cold. It started about a week ago and I can't shake it. My temperature was 100.2° last night and I've been getting the chills. The stuff I'm coughing up is starting to turn green.

Candidates for the COMLEX 2-PE cannot count on this happening in a standardized patient encounter. The standardized patients answer only the questions candidates ask.

LOGICAL SEQUENCE

An answer from a patient often leads the candidate to the next question. The candidate's role is to keep the patient on track while exploring the chief complaint and gaining sufficient information to obtain an accurate diagnosis. The stream of questioning can show the different thought processes behind the candidate's questions, as shown in Table 4–1.

In Table 4–1, the picture changes in the scenario depicted. The physician starts out thinking that the person may be an alcoholic and then recognizes the cardiovascular benefits of the patient's moderate alcohol consumption. However, if the physician discovers that the patient had been in rehab six times over the last 2 years for alcohol abuse, she would immediately return to the original opinion that drinking on a daily basis is not appropriate for this patient.

Candidates must never abandon a question for which they have received an incomplete answer. If a patient admits that he has had the same abdominal pain twice in the past, the candidate must ask about those past occurrences. When were they? How long did they last? How did they get better?

Table 4–1 Thought Process Behind Questions

	Dialogue	Physician's Thought Process
Candidate	Do you drink alcohol?	Social history screening
Patient	Yes.	Positive screen
Candidate	How often do you drink?	Follow-up question to positive
Patient	Every day.	Oh, my, that's a lot.
Candidate	How much do you drink in a day?	Quantifier
Patient	Oh, only one glass of wine a day.	Well, that's good for the heart.

COMPONENTS OF THE HISTORY OF PRESENT ILLNESS: CODIERS SMASH FM

This section provides the key to obtaining a complete yet concise history. Typically, physicians begin patient histories and allow the story to emerge in logical sequence based on the patient's answers to physician questions. The physician redirects when the patient strays too far away from the topic at hand and rephrases partially answered questions so that the patient can fill in any gaps.

The fact that there is no set sequence to questioning, however, does not mean that the physician's questions are not in a logical order. For example, when a patient presents with dizziness, one of the first questions the physician may ask is, "Describe what you mean by dizziness?" There are many other options for the next question: "When did you first have this dizziness? Have you ever had this before?"

Because there is no set sequence of questions, having a mnemonic to fall back on is valuable and can get candidates back on track should they get confused while taking the history. This mnemonic is CODIERS SMASH FM: chronology, onset, description/duration, intensity, exacerbating and remitting factors, symptoms associated, social history, medical history, allergies, surgical history, hospitalization history, family history, and medications. (See Table 4–2.)

Occasionally, candidates find that they are running out of questions, yet they still do not have a probable diagnosis. As discussed in Chapter 3, "Biomedical/Biomechanical Domain: Review of Patient Information and Introduction to the Patient," and as shown in Table 3–1, when candidates write the mnemonic along the left side of the data collection sheet or on scrap paper and fill in patient answers in the corresponding areas of the mnemonic, a brief glance at the paper can show them which areas have not yet been discussed.

For example, the first *M* in SMASH stands for medical history. The patient is a 20-year-old man who presents with chest pain while playing basketball. The pain is associated with shortness of breath. There is no radiation of the pain. Based on the history taken so far, the candidate includes spontaneous pneumothorax and musculoskeletal etiologies in the differential diagnosis. Because the patient is only 20 years old, the candidate may be tempted to skip asking about prior medical history, assuming none exists. When the candidate glances at the paper and sees the blank next to the *M* for medical history, he is prompted to ask, "Do you have any medical conditions?" The patient says, "I have Marfan's syndrome." Instantly, the candidate adds dissecting thoracic aortic aneurysm as a possible diagnosis and moves it up to the top of the differential as the most likely and most life threatening.

It may sound trite, but candidates should practice writing the mnemonic and what each letter stands for until they have memorized it. For the COMLEX 2-PE, once the beginning of the standardized patient timed encounter is announced, candidates should be able to write the mnemonic in less than 15 seconds.

CODIERS

CODIERS stands for chronology, onset, description/duration, intensity, exacerbating and remitting factors, and symptoms associated. Each component is discussed in more detail in the following subsections.

Table 4–2 CODIERS SMASH FM Mnemonic

Mnemonic	Overview	Specific Questions

C: Chronology:	Time frame showing the sequence of events	Have you ever had this BEFORE?
		
		  With a positive:
		
		  When was that?
		
		  When the first time you had it?
		
		  How often does it occur?
		
		  How long does it last?
		
		  Did you seek intervention?
		
		  Was there a prior diagnosis?
		
		  What was the prior treatment?
		
		  What was the prior outcome?
		
		How has it CHANGED?
		
		What was the order of symptoms?

O: Onset	Occurrence	When did the current symptoms start?
D: Description	Describe it	Can you DESCRIBE it to me? What does it FEEL like?
I: Intensity	Scale How bad is it?	On a scale from 1 to 10, how bad is the pain? How has the symptom affected your activities of daily living? What can't you do anymore?
E: Exacerbating factors		What makes it worse?
R: Remitting factors		What makes it better?
S: Symptoms associated	Concurrent findings	For a cold: Do you have fever, chills, runny nose, sinus pressure, headache, nasal congestion, sore throat, cough, etc.?
S: Social history	FED TACOS	Ask about food (diet), exercise, drugs, tobacco, alcohol, caffeine, occupation, and sexual history.
M: Medical history		Have you had any prior medical conditions (acute or chronic)? Which immunizations have you had? Have you had a mammogram (Health maintenance)?
A: Allergies		Food, environmental, drug—what happens?
S: Surgical history		What? When?
H: Hospitalization		What? Where? When?
F: Family history		Do any medical conditions run in the family? Mother, father, siblings, family tendencies?
M: Medications		What are the names, doses, and frequency of the medications you take?

Chronology/Onset

The mnemonic is a guide, not an absolute order in which questions should be asked. The acronym CODIERS groups together all of the aspects of the current complaint, whereas SMASH FM pertains to general medical and social history of the patient. Generally, the patient's story comes together more cohesively when physicians exhaust CODIERS prior to advancing to SMASH FM. This guideline,

COMLEX Level 2-PE Review Guide

however, should not interrupt the flow of the case. If a patient presents stating, "I think I'm having an allergic reaction to my medication!" likely the candidate's very first and most appropriate question would be, "Which medication?" Here, jumping to the last *M* in the mnemonic makes immense sense, and the candidate simply can return to CODIERS should logical flow dry up.

Timing of an event has many components represented by both C (chronology) and O (onset). Although chronology is the first letter in the mnemonic, typically physicians address onset first in clinical questioning:

> **Physician:** Miss Alyson, when did this start? (onset)
> **Patient:** About a week ago.

Chronology represents the time frame of the patient's symptoms and consists of three major areas outside of the onset:

- Prior history of the same complaint:

  > **Physician:** Have you ever had these headaches before?
  > **Patient:** No.
  > Or
  > **Patient:** Yes, I started getting them 2 years ago.

- How the complaint has changed since onset:

  > **Physician:** Has anything changed about the headaches?
  > **Patient:** Well, I used to get them once a month, but now it's once a week.

- Order of symptom presentation:

  > **Physician:** Which symptoms do you get first?
  > **Patient:** First, I see this fuzzy bright spot, and then I get a throbbing headache that makes me nauseated.

The chronology can be thought of as two separate time sequences. The first is from the onset, when the current complaint started ("About a week ago") until present, the time the candidate sees the patient. Within this period of time, the candidate needs to know how the complaint has changed since it started. For example, "The cough is keeping me up at night now" suggests progression of the symptom.

The second time sequence is only applicable if the patient has had similar episodes before. If the same complaint has occurred previously, candidates should thoroughly investigate it because exploring the prior history of the complaint can yield valuable clues. Candidates should find out the following information:

1. When the patient first had the symptoms
2. How often they occur
3. How long they last
4. Whether the patient sought intervention
5. Whether there is a prior diagnosis
6. What the prior treatment was
7. What the prior outcome was
8. Whether there has been any change in the pattern of occurrence

By using this line of questions, candidates might get a story along these lines:

> **Candidate:** Did you ever have this before? (chronology)
> **Patient:** Yes.
> **Candidate:** When was that?
> **Patient:** I started getting them 2 years ago.
> **Candidate:** Did you see anyone for it?
> **Patient:** I saw the family doctor we had before I moved here.
> **Candidate:** Did the doctor give you a diagnosis?

Patient: He said I was having migraine headaches.
Candidate: How did he treat you?
Patient: Well, he wanted to give me some pills, but I hate to take medicine. So, instead he gave me some paper that told me what to avoid that might be causing the headaches and a diary to keep track of what I ate.
Candidate: Did you find out what was causing them?
Patient: It did seem that I'd get the headaches more frequently when I had some wine.
Candidate: Did you cut out the wine to see if they went away?
Patient: Yeah, that seemed to work for a while.
Candidate: So, now you are getting them even though you're not drinking wine?
Patient: Well, Doc, I kind of slipped in watching the wine.

By exploring the prior history of the same complaint, not only did the candidate find the likely diagnosis, but also found out how to treat the patient. Instead of placing her on an expensive medication with possible side effects, trigger avoidance seems most appropriate.

Another case that emphasizes the need for thorough exploration of past similar complaints is a patient who walked into my office at 4:15 on a Friday afternoon. He was a 93-year-old man complaining of dizziness. Upon hearing this chief complaint with its huge range of possibilities and intensities of evaluation, a differential diagnosis alarm was set off inside my head. Thankfully, I did not abandon CODIERS SMASH FM. The questioning went like this:

Physician: Mr. Cook, what brings you in today?
Patient: I feel really dizzy. Almost falling down.
Physician: Have you ever had this before?
Patient: Yes, last year.
Physician: Did you see someone for it?
Patient: Yes.
Physician: What did they do for you?
Patient: They washed out my ears and fixed it just like that.

With baited anticipation I grabbed the otoscope and looked in at a plug of cerumen. Two minutes and a water evacuation later, he walked up and down the hall, stating the dizziness was completely gone. A thorough history often leads to a quick, definitive diagnosis and treatment.

Description/Duration

D should prompt the candidate to ask the patient to describe the symptoms. For example, if the patient presents complaining of pain, a specific description of the pain could easily alter or enhance the presumed diagnosis.

For example, a 78-year-old man presents with chest pain:

Candidate: Can you describe the chest pain?
Patient: It's like someone is sticking a knife in my chest.
Or
Patient: It feels like an elephant is sitting on my chest.

Which of these descriptive answers is more likely to represent an acute coronary syndrome? Candidates should always begin with the open-ended question as shown, and then move into the closed-ended questions should the case require.

Candidate: Can you describe the chest pain?
Patient: It hurts.
Candidate: Can you describe what you mean by "it hurts"?
Patient: It just feels bad.
Candidate: Would you say the pain is sharp, dull, achy, a pressure, burning . . . ?

Present the options slowly so that the patient can consider each as an accurate description of the pain.

The complaint of dizziness, in the previous case, provides another example of how description can help to narrow the diagnosis. When I asked Mr. Cook to describe his dizziness, he stated that he just felt off balance. Other clues could have altered the differential had he described his dizziness as a sensation of the room spinning around (vertigo, possible inner ear dysfunction), lightheadedness (possible anemia), or the room going dark (near syncope, possible cardiac arrhythmia).

Intensity

Not all histories include every component of CODIERS SMASH FM. For example, when a patent complains of a runny nose, the candidate need not find out the intensity of the problem, as in "How runny is it?" Some complaints lend themselves naturally to classic scales. A typical pain scale spans from 0 to 10, with 10 being the worst pain.

Intensity, however, can be judged by the effect the symptom has on the patient's activities of daily living (ADLs). For dizziness, candidates may be able to assign an imprecise intensity such as being so dizzy that the patient fell down, or so dizzy that the patient couldn't go to work that day.

Exacerbating and Remitting Factors

Questions about exacerbating or remitting factors are straightforward. However, a common error is to ask the patient both types of questions in one sentence:

Candidate: Does anything make your chest pain better or worse?
Patient: Spicy sauces and wine seem to make it worse.

Patients have a tendency to answer only the second half of the question; therefore, candidates should ask questions about exacerbating factors separate from remitting factors:

Candidate: Does anything make your chest pain better?
Patient: Antacids seem to tame it down a bit.
Candidate: Does anything else make it better?
Patient: It seems better if I don't eat before going to bed.
Candidate: Does anything make it worse?
Patient: Spicy sauces and wine seem to make it worse.
Candidate: Anything else?
Patient: Not that I noticed.

The candidate got a lot more information by asking each question separately but made another mistake by walking away from the line of questioning too quickly. For example, a more complete line of questioning in this case might be as follows:

Candidate: Does anything make your chest pain better?
Patient: Antacids seem to tame it down a bit.
Candidate: How often do you take antacids?
Patient: Every day.
Candidate: How many times a day?
Patient: Oh, four or five.
Candidate: What is the name of the antacid?
Patient: Whatever I get a hold of, mostly Tums.
Candidate: How many do you take at a time?
Patient: Oh, three or four.

That's a lot of antacid and may prompt the candidate to investigate more aggressively than if the patient took only one or two antacids once a week.

Symptoms Associated

Symptoms associated is another term for review of systems (ROS). This is an inventory of symptoms that the candidate develops as diagnoses enter the differential.

Diagnosis-Based Questioning

Candidates must ask for symptoms associated based on suspected diagnosis and not randomly, as in a generic review of system screen. This is frequently seen as students as everyone if they have fever, chills, nausea, or vomiting. Instead, as the candidate entertains thoughts of a possible diagnosis, he should ask symptoms related to that diagnosis to prove himself right or wrong.

For example, Mary Thomas is a 75-year-old woman who presents with shortness of breath (SOB). As the candidate works through CODIERS, he finds that Mary has had these symptoms before. The last occurrence was 1 year ago, when she was admitted to the hospital and treated for pneumonia. Immediately upon hearing this, the candidate considers another episode of pneumonia as a possible diagnosis. The candidate must ask himself, "What are the other signs and symptoms of pneumonia?" This prompts for inquiry about fever, chills, cough, sputum production, and chest pain.

However, many conditions can cause SOB. The next diagnosis that the candidate entertains is acute coronary syndrome. He then asks if the patient is experiencing any sweating, nausea, pain going into the arms or neck, and numbness or tingling.

As soon as a new possible diagnosis arises, candidates should ask the appropriate questions to prove it right or wrong. For example, the patient volunteers that she has a 40-pack year smoking history. The candidate adds acute exacerbation of chronic obstructive pulmonary disease (COPD) to the growing list of possible diagnoses and asks the patient if she can tell whether she has more problems getting the air in or getting it out. He also asks if she has been wheezing. When reviewing the patient's medications, the candidate learns that Mary takes both an ACE inhibitor and furosemide, a loop diuretic. These medications are commonly used to treat heart failure. Though the patient denies a history of heart failure, the candidate must add it to the differential. To rule it out, he must ask about difficulty breathing while lying flat (orthopnea), sudden shortness of breath while sleeping (paroxysmal nocturnal dyspnea), dyspnea on exertion, and peripheral edema.

Anatomy-Based Questioning

A second method for determining the appropriate symptoms associated should be based on anatomy and becomes practical to use in situations when the candidate is unsure of the diagnosis. After identifying the area of complaint, the candidate should work through organ involvement within the area.

Gwen is a 40-year-old woman who presents with right upper quadrant abdominal pain. While taking her history, the candidate considers cholelithiasis as a possible diagnosis and has, therefore, asked about exacerbation after eating fatty foods, radiation of the pain into the shoulder blade, and clay-colored stools. However, the candidate remains unconvinced that cholelithiasis is the final diagnosis.

The candidate can approach anatomy-based questioning by imagining an arrow passing straight through the patient's right upper quadrant directly from anterior to posterior. Consider which organs the arrow would touch as it passes through the body.

In this case, the first point of contact is the skin. The candidate must recall which conditions could cause pain of the skin in the right upper quadrant location. How about herpes zoster, shingles? The patient is not in the typical age group for this condition, but it is a possibility. The following questions address the symptoms associated with shingles:

- Did you have any tingling in the area before this started?
- Does the pain wrap around to the back?
- Do you have a rash or blisters?

The next points of contact are the subcutaneous tissues and the rib cage. Could this be a rib dysfunction or costochondritis?

- Do you have any pain with deep breaths?
- Does movement cause pain?
- Have you had any trauma?
- Do you have any shortness of breath?

Next the arrow would touch the parietal pleura. Is there an acute peritonitis such as could occur with a rupturing gallbladder?

- Do you have any fever?
- Nausea?
- Vomiting?
- Does it hurt to press in on your stomach?

The candidate continues by considering perforated viscous. Could this be a duodenal or gastric ulceration?

- Have you had any heart burn?
- Have you noticed any dark or sticky stools?

The transverse colon stretches across both upper quadrants. Could this be colitis?

- Do you have any changes to your stool?
- Diarrhea?
- Blood in your stools?
- Mucus?

The candidate has already considered the gallbladder, and next considers the rest of the biliary system: could this be distal obstruction, such as from a gallstone or pancreatic head cancer? Although the candidate has already asked questions about the gallbladder, she needs to find out whether there is pancreatic involvement:

- Have you had any weight loss?
- Night sweats?
- Lightheadedness?
- Left upper quadrant pain?
- Pain going into the back?

Next comes the liver. Is it possible the patient has acute hepatitis? Many symptoms about which the candidate has already asked overlap, such as clay-colored stools, nausea, and vomiting. The following questions are specific to the liver:

- Have you noticed any yellowness in your eyes or skin?
- Have you been in contact with anyone with hepatitis?
- Have you traveled recently?
- Have you had any exposure to blood or body fluids?
- Have you eaten any raw shellfish?

After the liver, the arrow would encounter the right kidney. Is this pyelonephritis? The candidate has already asked about fevers and back pain, but here are other questions pertaining to kidney dysfunction:

- Do you have any chills?
- Flank pain?
- Blood in your urine?
- Cloudy urine?
- Burning with urination?
- Foul-smelling urine?

Finally, the arrow would pass through the inferior lobe of the right lung. Could this be pneumonia?

- Do you have a cough?
- Sputum production?

Because the pain is anterior, renal and pneumonic etiologies are certainly lower in likelihood but can quickly be considered. Further, atypical etiologies exist such as a right upper quadrant appendix, but the candidate should stick with common and not atypical possibilities.

It is important for candidates to recognize that the symptoms associated are part of the history and are documented under the Subjective part of the note. (See Chapter 7, "SOAP Note Documentation.")

Table 4–3 contains several examples of ROS for each body area (it is far from exhaustive).

Table 4–3 Symptoms Associated: The Problem-Specific Review of Systems (ROS)

System	Symptoms
Constitution	Fever, chills, weight loss or gain, night sweats, fatigue
Eyes	Blurred or loss of vision, double vision, eye pain, injection, discharge, deviation
Ears, nose, mouth, and throat	Ear pain, discharge, hearing loss, epistaxis, nasal congestion, lesions, tooth pain, dysphagia, tinnitus, sore throat
Cardiovascular	Palpitations, chest pain, peripheral edema, claudication, irregular heart beats, murmur
Respiratory	Shortness of breath, orthopnea, dyspnea on exertion, coughing, wheezing, chest pain, paroxysmal nocturnal dyspnea, hemoptysis
Gastrointestinal	Dyspepsia, nausea, vomiting, diarrhea, constipation, eructation, bloating, hematemesis, hematochezia, abdominal pain, change in caliber of the stools, bright red blood per rectum, melena
Genitourinary	Hesitancy, flank pain, dysuria, hematuria, urgency, frequency, decrease in force of stream, vaginal or penile discharge, dyspareunia, hematospermia
Musculoskeletal	Arthralgia, myalgia, boney deformity, weakness
Integumentary/breast	Changes in pigmentation or texture, rashes, lesions, pruritus, hair loss or change in hair texture, nail changes, dimpling
Neurologic	Facial asymmetry, memory loss, paresthesias, weakness, slurred speech, imbalance, changes in gait, dysphagia
Psychiatric	Depression, suicidal or homicidal ideation, anxiety, hallucinations
Endocrine	Polyuria, polyphagia, polydipsia, heat or cold intolerances
Hematologic/lymphatic	Easy bruising or bleeding, anemia, transfusion history, syncope, lymphadenopathy
Allergic/immunologic	Allergies, recurrent infections

SMASH FM

SMASH FM represents the general medical and social history of the patient. Again, logical flow and following clues from the patient's answers can lead candidates to the next appropriate question. For example, SMASH FM puts medications at the end. Candidates will likely find themselves asking about medications much earlier in the patient interview when a historical clue prompts this line of questioning. The patient interview is fluid, meaning that candidates will find themselves jotting down answers and skipping back and forth between CODIERS and SMASH FM as the story unfolds. Once this logical flow ebbs, candidates can glance at their paper to see where gaps in the mnemonic need to be filled in. By filling in the gaps, candidates can complete a most detailed history.

Social History

This *S* stands for social history. To thoroughly assess social history, candidates can write a second mnemonic on their paper horizontally across from the first *S* in SMASH: FED TACOS. (See Figure 4–1.) FED TACOS stands for food, exercise, drugs, tobacco, alcohol, caffeine, occupation, and sexual history.

The candidate should glance at the FED TACOS social history mnemonic and consider whether the questioning is appropriate for the problem at hand. For example, if a 27-year-old male roofer presents with shoulder pain that resulted from grabbing a bucket full of nails as it slid off a roof, the candidate need not inquire about his diet represented by *F* for food.

However, his E (exercise) habits might indeed be very important as would his O (occupation). How is this injury going to affect his ability to play on the softball team and when will he be able to return to work?

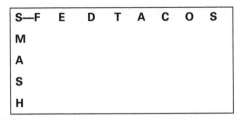

Figure 4–1 Social History Note Taking: FED TACOS

The FED TACOS mnemonic is shown in Table 4–4.

In obtaining the social history, candidates should begin with the least sensitive questions first and advance into the more sensitive areas. For example, to take a history from Alyson Roth, a 16-year-old girl with ear pain: although she presents only for ear pain, it is important to perform the social history screen. Approaching Alyson, the candidate observes that she appears to be an appropriate weight, so he discards the food and exercise questions, although some candidates choose to ask questions in each area of the social history regardless. Candidates must remember that they have only 14 minutes for each case in the exam.

Next in the mnemonic is *D* for drugs. The defenses of this adolescent patient may fly up if the next question the candidate asks her is, "Do you use any drugs?" First, she probably will not see any association between her ear pain and that question and may feel that the candidate is accusing her of something.

So, it is helpful for candidates to begin with the least offensive question in the drugs area such as about caffeine use, followed by questions about tobacco, alcohol, and then drugs. The candidate's approach should be matter of fact and he might even begin with an explanation of why he is asking these questions:

> **Candidate:** Alyson, next I'm going to take a social history from you. I ask the same questions of everyone. How much caffeine is in your diet including coffee, pop, and chocolate?
> **Patient:** I drink a pop or two a day, but it's decaffeinated.
> **Candidate:** Do you use any tobacco?
> **Patient:** I smoke a little.
> **Candidate:** How much is a little?
> **Patient:** One or two cigarettes a day.
> **Candidate:** Only one or two?
> **Patient:** Yes. I never buy them. My friends all smoke, so when they drive me to school they give me a cigarette and then they give me one on the way home too.
> **Candidate:** How long have you been doing that?
> **Patient:** Just this year.
> **Candidate:** Do you drink any alcohol?
> **Patient:** No.
> **Candidate:** Do you use any street drugs or prescription drugs?
> **Patient:** Nope.

By starting with the most benign questions such as about caffeine, the candidate is more likely to get honest answers as he progresses because the patient feels that these are just screening questions and not accusations. Later, the candidate can return to the issue of smoking and the need for smoking cessation as part of the plan.

The *O* for occupation should be screened for two primary reasons. First, the candidate must determine whether the chief complaint is directly related to the patient's occupation. The candidate can assume that Alyson, a 16-year-old female, is a student and does not work, or he can doubt that her occupation has anything to do with her ear pain. However, he might ask about her occupation and find that she is a life guard. He might have also picked this up under exercise. A little further questioning about her life guard duties reveals that after she finishes her shift at the pool, she soaks in the hot tub for an hour, and yes, she puts her head under the water. The candidate should now consider

Table 4–4 Social History Mnemonic: FED TACOS

Mnemonic	Examples of Pertinence

F: Food	Nutritional balance—weight loss
	Restrictions—Sodium in hypertension
	               Carbohydrates in diabetes
	               Cholesterol in coronary artery disease
	               Fats in cholelithiasis

E: Exercise	Obesity Cardiac rehabilitation Musculoskeletal injury Health maintenance
D: Drugs	Street drugs—recreational use Prescription drug abuse—chronic pain syndromes
T: Tobacco	Smoking—Shortness of breath Smokeless tobacco (chewing tobacco)—mouth lesions
A: Alcohol	Abdominal pain—pancreatitis Cough and shortness of breath—aspiration pneumonia Depression—abuse Dyspepsia—reflux esophagitis
C: Caffeine	Coffee, tea, pop, chocolate—tachycardia, insomnia

O: Occupation	Etiologies
	    Shortness of breath—asbestosis
	    Rash—contact dermatitis
	Limitations—When can the patient return to work?

S: Sexual History	Obstetrical history
	    Menarche
	    Menopause
	    Menstruation
	FDLNMP—First day of last normal menstrual period
	Sexually transmitted diseases
	Pregnancy planning and prevention

Pseudomonas otitis externa as a possible cause. Perhaps a question about occupation was appropriate to ask after all.

The second reason to review the occupation comes into play during development of the plan of treatment. For example, physicians cannot send a daycare worker back to work with pinkeye until the infection has cleared. Knowing about the patient's occupation allows the physician to assess whether restrictions must be placed on working.

The final *S* in FED TACOS, which stands for sexual history, will likely be the most skipped area of questioning. If Mrs. Dunley, an 83-year-old woman, presents with a cough, the candidate need not ask her whether she is sexually active. However, if the same patient presents with vaginal discharge, it is an appropriate question.

Very frequently, the only sexual history question pertinent to the case is inquiring about the patient's first day of last menstrual period (FDLMP) because this should be a consideration in both diagnostics and treatment options. Again, with a complaint of cough, you needn't ask Mrs. Dunley when her last period was.

Medical History

The first *M* in SMASH FM stands for medical history. This should include acute and chronic medical conditions, injuries, and immunizations as appropriate.

Some ways to pose these questions are as follows:

- Do you have any medical conditions?
- Have you been treated for any medical issues in the past?
- Are you being treated for any medical problems?
- Have you had any injuries?
- Are your immunizations up-to-date?

Candidates may also have to ask about specific immunizations as cases present:

- When was your last tetanus shot?
- Did you get the flu shot this year?

Allergies

Allergy history should investigate three categories of allergies: foods, drugs, and environmental allergies. In addition, it is not enough to know that the patient has an allergy to something, the candidate must also find out what his or her reaction is:

> **Candidate:** Do you have any food allergies?
> **Patient:** Yes, I'm allergic to bananas.
> **Candidate:** What happens?
> **Patient:** I can't breathe.

This represents a true anaphylactic reaction, and the candidate must ensure that the patient has an up-to-date prescription for an epinephrine auto injector (EpiPen).

> **Candidate:** Are you allergic to any medications?
> **Patient:** Penicillin.
> **Candidate:** What happens?
> **Patient:** I'm not sure. My mother just always told me never to take it.

Here, the candidate cannot be sure whether the patient has a true allergy or not. The candidate could avoid the use of penicillin as a first line, but if limited options remained, the candidate could test the patient to see whether a true penicillin allergy exists.

> **Candidate:** Are you allergic to any medications?
> **Patient:** Aspirin.
> **Candidate:** What happens?
> **Patient:** It upsets my stomach.

This is not a true allergic reaction, but rather an adverse reaction. Perhaps the patient has only tried non-enteric-coated aspirin at higher doses. Because he has diabetes, a trial of low-dose, enteric-coated aspirin would be appropriate.

Surgical History

Under surgical history, candidates ask what was done and when it was performed. If appropriate, the candidate can go into more specific detail such as the symptoms prompting the need for surgery, complications, and the outcome.

For example, Elaine Angle, a 32-year-old woman, presents with abdominal pain and fever:

> **Candidate:** Have you had any prior surgeries?
> **Patient:** Yes.
> **Candidate:** What did you have done?
> **Patient:** I had my appendix taken out.
> **Candidate:** When was that?
> **Patient:** About 10 years ago.

The candidate knows that the current complaint is not related to Elaine's appendix. With the same patient the candidate might go further:

> **Candidate:** Have you had any other prior surgeries?
> **Patient:** Yes.
> **Candidate:** What did you have done?
> **Patient:** I just had a baby.
> **Candidate:** When was that?
> **Patient:** About 5 days ago.
> **Candidate:** Was it a vaginal delivery or caesarian section?
> **Patient:** Vaginal.

Here, the candidate must consider complications of the delivery including retained placenta.

Hospitalization History

For hospitalization history, besides the approximate dates, candidates should inquire as to the reason, treatments incurred, and outcomes.

Family History

In the 14-minute exam encounter, candidates must be wary of spending too much time in the family history area. They should base their questioning broadly, and then focus as appropriate.

> **Candidate:** Do any medical conditions run in the family?

For example, a 42-year-old woman, Mrs. Green, presents with polyuria without dysuria. The candidate notes her body habitus shows truncal obesity.

> **Candidate:** Mrs. Green, does anyone in your family have diabetes or sugar problems?

Also under family history candidates must consider contacts the patient may have had with others who have the same symptoms. For example, Lyncean, a 24-year-old medical student, presents with vomiting and diarrhea:

> **Candidate:** Does anyone in your family or anyone else you've been in contact with have the same symptoms?
> **Patient:** Yes. I went out to eat with several of my friends last evening. Jen has the same thing.
> **Candidate:** Did you eat the same things?
> **Patient:** We had different entrées, but we both had fried rice.
> **Candidate:** Did anyone else eat the rice and not get sick?
> **Patient:** I don't think anyone else had it.

If a patient presents for an acute musculoskeletal history, it would be much more appropriate to minimize the family history and focus on more high-yield data such as those found elsewhere in the history.

Medications

Finally, the last *M* in SMASH FM stands for medications. Candidates must know the name of each medication and the dose and frequency that the patient has been taking it. They should be sure to include prescription medications, over-the-counter medications, herbs, and vitamins as appropriate.

For example, Willie Maket, a 78-year-old farmer, presents with knee pain.

> **Candidate:** Are you on any medications?
> **Patient:** No. I don't like to take medications.
> **Candidate:** Did you take anything to try to make it better?
> **Patient:** I took some ibuprofen. It didn't do a thing.
> **Candidate:** How much did you take?
> **Patient:** Two little brown pills.
> **Candidate:** How often did you take them?
> **Patient:** Just that once. Like I said, they didn't do much for it.
> **Candidate:** When did you take them?
> **Patient:** A couple of days ago.

This frequency of dosing does not represent a therapeutic failure, but rather a failure to treat at appropriate doses. It does not exclude nonsteroidals as a treatment option.

Candidates are now armed with the two mnemonics that can guide them through a thorough collection of data and help them master a major component of the Biomedical/Biomechanical domain. Candidates should memorize these mnemonics and know what each letter represents.

Biomedical/Biomechanical Domain: Physical Examination

After completing the history-taking component, the candidate should have formed a differential diagnosis. (Differential diagnoses are discussed in detail in Chapter 6, "Biomedical/Biomechanical Domain: Assessment and Plan.") Although some cases require no examination—such as cases that focus on patient education, for example, when a patient presents to inquire about colonoscopy because his brother was just diagnosed with colon cancer or a patient seeks advice on pregnancy planning—most of the standard patient encounters for the COMLEX 2-PE require candidates to perform a problem-specific physical examination. With the limited time frame of 14 minutes per case, the examination must focus on the principal complaints and diagnoses that the candidate is considering.

There are two methods to consider when approaching the examination. The recommended approach is a head-to-toe approach in which the candidate considers each system and whether examination of that system has bearing on the case. The second method is for the candidate to approach the area of complaint first, and then spread the examination to adjacent areas. Both are discussed in detail in this chapter.

Candidates must approach each encounter as if they are encountering a real patient and accept the physical examination findings for what they are. If the standardized patient has a murmur, candidates are expected to identify it during the exam. Candidates must not simply go through the motions of auscultating the heart in the four valvular areas, but must truly listen for and document abnormal findings.

Likewise, if a patient presents with knee trauma and the candidates identifies ecchymosis during inspection, the candidate shouldn't say, "That looks too painful to touch." Candidates should use range-of-motion techniques to identify limitations and palpatory techniques to localize the area of trauma and make a precise diagnosis.

THE PATIENT DATA SHEET

Regardless of which method of examination the candidate chooses to use, the examination begins outside the room with the patient data sheet and a review of the vital signs. The following are sample patient data such as is provided on the patient data sheet:

CC: A 68 y/o male presents with a cough

Blood pressure: 168/92

Respirations: 28 bpm

Pulse: 120 bpm

Temperature: 102.2°F

Weight: 168 lbs

Height: 5'11"

Candidates should review the vital signs before entering the room. Temperature, weight, and height measures never need to be repeated; however, measures of abnormal blood pressures, respirations, and pulse rates should be repeated. Candidates should accept the vital signs provided for the standardized patient as true findings. In this case, the screening blood pressure must be addressed. If the candidate recognizes the blood pressure is elevated at 168/92 mm HG on the screening sheet, and repeats the blood pressure measurement to find it is now 120/60, he cannot state that the first reading was an error. Regardless of whether the patient is known to have hypertension or this is a new finding of elevated blood pressure, the candidate must accept the abnormal screening pressure as real and plan for follow-up return visits to recheck the blood pressure on two additional separate occasions.

Candidates should repeat vital signs falling outside of normal ranges as listed below:

- Systolic blood pressure > 130
- Diastolic blood pressure > 80
- Pulse < 60 beats per minute
- Pulse > 100 beats per minute
- Respirations < 12 breaths per minute
- Respirations > 20 breaths per minute

To prompt themselves to repeat abnormal vital signs, candidates can circle, star, or in some other fashion draw attention to the abnormal vital sign on the patient data sheet as they begin the physical examination. (See Figure 5–1.)

BEGINNING THE EXAMINATION

Before they begin the examination, candidates should consider the Humanistic domain as discussed in Chapter 2 and be sure the address its components throughout the exam. After they have finished their initial questioning, candidates can follow these guidelines:

- Advise the patient that they are about to start the physical examination.
- Ask the patient for permission to do so.
- Rewash their hands if they have contaminated themselves in any way.
- Ask for permission to expose areas of examination.
- Re-cover the areas of examination as soon as permissible.
- Assist the patient in position changes no matter what the age of the patient.
- Drape the patient from the waist down with the sheet provided if they will be exposing the abdomen.
- Slide the sheet upward to examine the lower extremities, keeping the groin covered at all times.

CC	: A 68 y/o male presents with a cough
Blood pressure	: 168/92
Respirations	: 28 bpm
Pulse	: 120 bpm
Temperature	: 102.2 degrees F
Weight	: 168 lbs
Height	: 5'11"

Figure 5–1 How to Mark an Abnormal Vital Sign

COMPARISON OF EXAMINATION METHODS

The Head-to-Toe method of examination is recommended over the Target approach. Each is compared here.

Case Scenario

For the following comparison of examination methods, this case scenario is used: A 78-year-old man with history of hypertension, hyperlipidemia, and coronary artery disease status post myocardial infarction × 2 with known history of cardiomyopathy presents with progressive shortness of breath. During the history taking, the candidate finds that he has not been following his diet, he has been using salt liberally, and he has stopped taking his diuretic because it makes him urinate too frequently. The patient has a cough, dyspnea on exertion, orthopnea, and peripheral edema with a 15-pound weight gain since his last visit. He admits to chest pain, but localizes it to the rib cage bilaterally, which he attributes to his persistent cough. He denies fever, chills, sputum production, nausea, vomiting, pain in the neck or arm, paresthesias, or diaphoresis. The candidate's primary diagnosis is heart failure. How should the candidate approach the examination? (See Figure 5–2.)

Recommended Head-to-Toe Method of Examination

The candidate has already reviewed the vital signs on the patient data sheet, noting tachypnea and a normal temperature. The candidate would only repeat the respiratory rate measure because the blood pressure and pulse rate are within normal ranges. The candidate would not repeat the weight and would accept the reading as accurate. Reviewing and repeating the vitals takes less than 1 minute.

Taking the patient's history gives the candidate ample opportunity to perform a general assessment and note the patient's level of alertness, any distress including obvious cyanosis, pallor or labored breathing, position of comfort, body habitus, and his general state of self-care.

When candidates approach the examination using the head-to-toe method, they must briefly scan the body system and ask themselves whether examining it contributes to the proposed diagnosis, a diagnosis of heart failure in this case. Candidates begin at the top of the body:

- Head: No contribution to heart failure. Do not examine. Move to the next area.
- Eyes: No contribution. Do not examine. Move to the next area.
- Ears: No contribution. Do not examine. Move to the next area.
- Nose: No contribution. Do not examine. Move to the next area.
- Mouth: No contribution. Do not examine. Move to the next area.

If the patient had admitted to symptoms of an upper respiratory infection (URI), it would have been appropriate for the candidate to perform a head, eye, ear, nose, and throat (HEENT) exam. However, in this case, because he does not have URI symptoms and the HEENT exam would not elicit signs of heart failure, no HEENT exam is indicated. Perhaps the candidate might find hypertensive

```
CC              : A 78 y/o male presents with shortness of breath
Blood pressure : 110/62
Respirations    : 28 bpm
Pulse           : 90 bpm          ዋ
Temperature     : 98.2 degrees F
Weight          : 230 lbs
Height          : 5'11"
```

Figure 5–2 Heart Failure

retinopathy; however, the candidate already knows that the patient has a known history of hypertension. In this acute case, signs of hypertension do not affect the immediate treatment plan and should therefore not be evaluated immediately. If the candidate completes the examination, provides a diagnosis and treatment plan, and still has time left over, she could always go back and perform the ophthalmoscopic examination.

The candidate then continues moving from head to toe with the examination:

- Neck: Here, the candidate can make an association with heart failure because patients often have jugular venous distension. Further, the patient is known to have atherosclerosis with a history of myocardial infarction. Auscultation of the carotids is appropriate to assess for carotid bruits. For the neck, the candidate should follow the proper order of examination:
  - Inspection:
    - Jugular venous distention (JVD)
    - Accessory muscle use
    - Position of the trachea
  - Auscultation: Carotid bruits
  - Palpation: None indicated. Had the patient presented with symptoms of heart failure and was found to have a tachyarrhythmia, palpation of the thyroid would be appropriate.
  - Percussion: None indicated

Techniques of examination include inspection, auscultation, palpation, and percussion. The typical order of applying these techniques had been inspection, percussion, palpation, and then auscultation. However, there are noted exceptions to the rule, the neck should be auscultated prior to palpation to avoid compressing stenotic carotid arteries, and auscultation should precede palpation of the abdomen to avoid changing the pattern of bowel sounds which could occur if the abdomen is palpated prior to auscultation.

Merrine, a first-year medical student then presented this argument: Is there any system that would be adversely affected if auscultated prior to palpation, and if not, why remember an order of examination that requires adjustments under certain conditions? Why not use an order that does not have exceptions? Being unable to find contraindications to auscultation prior to palpation in any systems, I currently recommend the order: inspection, auscultation, palpation, and percussion.

Inspection of the neck for JVD with auscultation of the carotids takes less than 30 seconds, somewhat more time if the candidate has to make position changes to measure for JVD at 30° incline. Next, the candidate continues the caudad drift.

Now the candidate is at the heart of the matter, no pun intended. The next two systems are the greatest contributors to the proposed diagnosis of heart failure. The examination should become focused and detailed, incorporating all four components of examination techniques.

- Respiratory:
  - Inspection:
    - Appropriate exposure of the thorax
      - Ask the patient to lower the gown as appropriate.
      - Help the patient to do so.
      - Replace the gown as soon as possible to preserve dignity.
    - Accessory muscle use
    - Intercostal retractions
    - Anterior posterior/lateral (AP/lat) ratio
  - Auscultation:
    - Auscultation should be performed on bare skin, never on any clothing.
    - The candidate should advise the patient to take deep breaths in and out through the mouth.
    - The candidate should auscultate through complete inspiration and expiration and should not move the stethoscope prior to the end of complete expiration, such as when end expiratory wheezes would be expected.
    - The candidate should use symmetrical comparison, anterior right apex to anterior left apex, not down the anterior right side, and then down the anterior left side.

- The candidate should auscultate in two positions bilaterally anteriorly with one at the apex above the clavicle, two areas laterally, and three areas posteriorly.
  - Palpation:
    - Reproduction of tenderness with the complaint of rib pain with coughing
    - Evaluation for viscerosomatic findings and rib dysfunction
    - Tactile fremitus: Symmetrical approach at same levels as auscultation
  - Percussion:
    - Assessing for dullness of the bases
    - Assessing for areas of consolidation: Symmetrical approach at same levels as auscultation
  - Special techniques: These should be performed only if abnormalities are found with auscultation, palpation, or percussion.
    - Egophony
    - Whispered pectoriloquy
    - Bronchophony

By advancing through the examination techniques in order, candidates can perform only those that are necessary. For example, in this patient, the candidate first inspects the chest. Moving to auscultation, she finds the lungs are perfectly clear. All areas of auscultation show that breath sounds are full and clear without adventitious sounds or diminished breath sounds in the bases. Because this is one of the primary areas of concern in this case scenario with a chief complaint of shortness of breath, the candidate continues through palpation and percussion. If these are negative, no special testing is required such as egophony tactile fremitus.

The lung examination takes 90 seconds.

- Cardiac:
  - Inspection:
    - Assist the patient to the supine position
    - Precordial heave
    - Visible point of maximal impulse (PMI)
  - Auscultation:
    - Four valvular areas: Aortic, pulmonic, tricuspid, and mitral
    - Special positions only if murmur found:
      - Valsalva
      - Left lateral decubitus
      - Leaning forward
  - Palpation:
    - Point of maximal impulse (PMI)
    - Thrill:
      - Four valvular areas
      - Only if murmur found

The cardiac exam takes only 20 seconds.

- Abdomen:
  - Inspection:
    - Appropriately drape the patient's lower extremities with a sheet
    - Appropriate exposure
    - Distention/ascites
  - Auscultation: Consider atherosclerotic disease
    - Aortic bruit
  - Palpation:
    - Fluid wave: Only if ascites present
    - Consider estimation of diameter of the aorta
  - Percussion:
    - Liver span
    - Shifting dullness: Only if ascites present

- Special testing:
  - Hepatojugular reflex

The abdominal exam takes 30 seconds.

- Extremities:
  - Inspection:
    - Edema
    - Cyanosis

Examination of the extremities takes 10 seconds.

- Musculoskeletal: No contribution. Do not examine. Move to the next area.
- Neurologic: The candidate accessed the patient's level of alertness previously during history taking. No contribution. Do not examine. Move to the next area.
- Osteopathic: Assessed concurrently with other system exams as earlier.

When the candidate has completed the examination, she can assist the patient back to a seated position. The total time elapsed is summarized in Table 5–1.

At this point, the candidate has completed the physical examination portion of a very complex encounter, doing so in just a little more than 4 minutes. Most of the patient encounters are much more limited in complexity and require even less time for the examination.

The Target Method

The target approach incorporates a targeted area examination technique. Many medical students prefer this technique; however, it is likely that the standardized patients are trained to expect the candidate to perform the examination using the recommended head-to-toe method.

When the candidate approaches the patient with suspected heart failure in this case scenario using the target method, the examination again begins with reassessment of vitals, if abnormal, and the general assessment.

From this point, however, the candidate can imagine placing a target over the area of primary concern. The bull's eye of the target in a case of suspected heart failure is the heart. This target area is also called the absolute area—the area that absolutely needs to be examined. For example, the absolute area is the heart in heart failure, the throat in a patient with a sore throat, and the shoulder in a patient with shoulder pain. From the bull's eye, the candidate then spreads the examination outward to adjacent organ systems like the rings on a target (see Figure 5–3).

In this case, the candidate then moves laterally to the first ring of the target to examine the lungs. The lungs are areas in proximity to the heart, or areas adjacent to the bull's eye. Other areas adjacent to the heart might move the examination upward to the neck, which is closely associated with the heart through vasculature.

Finally, the candidate examines the second ring of associated areas, which are those that are related to the proposed diagnosis by system or disease. In consideration of the typical signs of heart failure, the candidate examines the abdomen for ascites and hepatomegaly, and the extremities for edema and assessment of peripheral pulses.

Table 5–1 Sample Elapsed Examination Time

System	Elapsed time
Vital signs	1 minute
Neck	20 seconds
Lungs	2 minutes
Heart	20 seconds
Abdomen	30 seconds
Extremities	10 seconds
Total Time Elapsed	4 minutes and 20 seconds

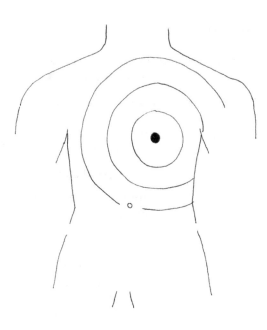

Figure 5–3 Bull's Eye

A summary of the target method is as follows:

- Bull's eye: Absolute area—cardiac exam
- First ring: Adjacent systems and structures
  - Respiratory exam
  - Neck exam
- Second ring: Associated areas
  - Abdominal exam
  - Extremities exam

PROHIBITED EXAMINATIONS

Sensitive examinations such as genital, rectal, female breast, and internal pelvic exams are *never* performed on the standardized patient. If any of these exams are indicated, candidates can advise the standardized patient of such and write the intention to perform the exam in the Plan section of the SOAP note, stating the exam should have been included. In addition, to protect the standardized patient, no corneal reflex exams are to be performed.[1p5]

TIPS FOR PHYSICAL EXAMINATION BY SYSTEM

As they move further into their years of clinical experience, it is common for practitioners to begin to take shortcuts in examination, such as placing the stethoscope centrally over the heart and listening only in that one position instead of over the four valvular areas of auscultation. This leads to incomplete and sloppy examination such as in this example.

- Auscultation of the lungs in a patient with a cough: The candidate does a screening auscultation that includes only one area anteriorly and two areas posteriorly, with no lateral auscultation. Standards for examination require that lung auscultation includes two positions bilaterally anteriorly, with one at the apex above the clavicle, two areas laterally, and three areas posteriorly.

In addition, practitioners sometimes begin to go through the motions without actually paying attention to what they are doing. They might listen to the heart and then move on in the exam, only to find themselves thinking, "Wait a minute. I think I heard something." When they return to the area, they find a low-grade murmur. Candidates must remember that the standardized patients they examine have true pathology. If the standardized patient has a murmur, candidates are expected to detect it in the examination. So, candidates must perform the examination on the patient to search for pathology. Missing true pathology will decrease the performance score.

- Auscultation of the lungs in a patient with a cough: The standardized patient has a true history of pulmonary fibrosis and has basilar crackles that are missed on auscultation.
- Inspection of the throat in a patient with sore throat: The candidate does not use a light source or tongue blade and fails to notice that the patient has had his uvula removed for sleep apnea.

Follow the proper examination techniques and avoid shortcuts.

➤ This symbol denotes areas where inappropriate examination techniques are commonly used and which shortcuts should be avoided.

Vital Signs

Again, candidates should accept the vital signs on the patient data sheet as correct. However, if an abnormality is documented, it behooves the candidate to recheck abnormalities of the pulse, respirations, and blood pressures. Measurement of the blood pressure is often a rushed examination. Proper technique is listed in Table 5–2. Following this proper technique, candidates can complete an accurate blood pressure in about 30 seconds.

Integumentary Exam

Table 5–2 Proper Blood Pressure Technique

1	Ask patient if there are any restrictions to taking a BP in either arm.
2	Ask patient about nicotine/caffeine in the last 30 minutes.
3	▶ Bare arm.
4	Locate the brachial artery by palpation.
5	Apply cuff with artery marker overlying brachial artery on bare skin.
6	Apply cuff 2.5 cm proximal to antecubital fossa with correct side down.
7	Ensure appropriately sized cuff by evaluating range markers.
8	Inflate while palpating radial artery, note disappearance.
9	Deflate and reinflate to 20 mm Hg above disappearance.
10	Auscultate brachial artery.
11	Deflate cuff at a rate of 2–3 mm per second.
12	Repeat in other arm if appropriate.

➤ The rule here is simply about exposing the skin properly.

Skin cannot be examined through clothing. Toenails cannot be examined through shoes. Again, candidates must remember to ask permission to perform the exam and obtain exposure, and then should re-cover the patient as soon as examination in the area is completed.

Following are guidelines and techniques for how candidates should perform the rest of the physical exam:

HEENT Exam

- Ears
  - Otoscopic exam
    - Invert the otoscope.
      - ➤ Distend the 5th digit to protect the tympanic membrane should the patient suddenly rotate the head.

- Straighten the canal by pulling:
  - Up, back, and out for an adult
  - Down, back, and out for a child
  - Hearing tests
    - Rhinne
      - Strike the tuning fork and place the handle on the mastoid process.
      - Ensure that the patient can hear it and advise the patient to say when he or she no longer can hear it.
      - When the patient can no longer hear the tone, without restriking, rotate the tines in front of the external ear and ask the patient if he or she can hear it again.
      - If the patient can hear it, this means air conduction (AC) is greater than bone conduction (BC), which suggests either a normal exam or a sensorineural hearing loss in that ear.
      - If the patient cannot hear it, then BC > AC, reflecting either a conductive loss in the ear being tested or a sensorineural loss in the opposite ear.
- Visual acuity: When testing vision, candidates should be sure to cover each eye. individually.
- Extra-ocular movements fields
  - Have the patient focus on finger or penlight held midline at level of eyes
  - Advise the patient to follow the object with the eyes only, holding the head still
  - Move the object through a full range of motion, typically in an H formation
  - Return to the central position and move the object toward the patient to check accommodation
- Pupillary reaction: Check both direct and consensual reaction.
- Ophthalmoscopic exam
  - Candidates *must not* turn off the lights of the exam room because the video reviewers will not be able to see what is occurring.
  - ➤ Candidates should use their right eye to exam the patient's right eye and their left eye to examine the patient's left eye.
- Mouth
  - ➤ Use a light source. Candidates cannot properly see inside the mouth without light.
  - ➤ Use a tongue blade. Move the buccal mucosa and lips for a thorough examination.
  - Candidates may not perform a gag reflex. If one is indicated, document that it should be performed in the SOAP note.

Neck Exam
- ➤ Carotids: Auscultate the carotids prior to palpation.
- Thyroid
  - Perform the exam while standing behind the patient.
  - Ask the patient to swallow while palpating the lobes.

Respiratory Exam
- Inspection:
  - Properly expose the chest—ask permission to do so first.
  - Re-cover the patient as soon as possible.
- Auscultation:
  - Instruct the patient to take deep breaths, in and out, through the mouth.
  - ➤ Auscultate on bare skin.
  - ➤ Auscultate through complete inspiration and expiration prior to moving to the next area of auscultation.
  - ➤ Use a symmetrical approach, examining the same level on each side, such as the right apex to the left apex, instead of down the right side, and then down the left.
  - ➤ Minimal areas of examination
  - Two levels anteriorly with one level above the clavicle at the apex
  - Two levels laterally

- ○ Three levels posteriorly with the superior-level auscultation medial off of the scapula and moving laterally as moving caudate
- Percussion:
  - ➤ Just as in auscultation, use a symmetrical approach, examining the same level on each side, such as the right apex to the left apex, instead of down the right side, and then down the left.

Cardiac Exam

- Inspection:
  - ○ Properly expose the precordium after asking permission to do so.
  - ○ Re-cover the patient as soon as possible.
  - ○ If examining in the supine position, assist the patient with the position change.
- Auscultation:
  - ➤ Auscultate on bare skin
  - ➤ At each valvular area:
    - ▪ Aortic—second intercostal space, right sternal border
    - ▪ Pulmonic—second intercostal space, left sternal border
    - ▪ Tricuspid—4th or 5th intercostal space, left sternal border
    - ▪ Mitral—4th or 5th intercostal space, left midclavicular line
  - ○ Candidates may ask female patients to lift the left breast to provide access to the tricuspid and mitral valves.

Abdominal Exam

- ➤ Assist the patient into the supine position.
- ➤ Cover the lower groin and legs with the sheet provided.
- Raise the gown to provide exposure of the abdomen, leaving the sheet covering the pelvis and lower extremities.
- Auscultate in all four quadrants.
- Palpation:
  - ○ Watch the patient's face during the examination.
  - ○ Stop or reduce pressure if the patient indicates that the exam is "a little rough" or is otherwise uncomfortable.
  - ○ Begin with a one-handed light palpation technique.
  - ○ Continue with the two-handed deeper palpation technique.

Vascular Exam

- Compare pulses bilaterally such as radial to radial, brachial to brachial, and so forth.
- Perform capillary refill bilaterally on both upper and lower extremities, removing the patient's shoes and socks.

Osteopathic Musculoskeletal Examination

- Inspection should include range of motion of each joint involved in the case.
- Compare bilaterally moving both joints through full active range of motion.
- Perform passive range of motion if any limitation to active range of motion is detected.
- Palpation:
  - ○ Tissue texture changes
  - ○ Chapman points, viscerosomatic reflexes
  - ○ Somatic dysfunction

Neurologic Examination

- Muscle strength testing: Compare bilaterally
- Sensory examination:
  - ○ Compare dermatomal nerve roots bilaterally.
  - ○ Use sharp/dull and light touch techniques.

- Reflexes:
  - ➤ Compare bilaterally: bicep to bicep, tricep to tricep, brachioradialis to brachioradialis, patella to patella, and Achilles to Achilles
  - ○ Have the muscle being tested relaxed because a partially contracted muscle will not demonstrate a proper reflex.
  - ○ Strike with a hinged wrist technique at the appropriate location.
  - ○ Provide patient distraction if reflexes are difficult to obtain, such as having the patient abduct the elbows, hook the fingers of each hand together while pulling apart and looking at the ceiling.

Sensitive Exams: Genital, Breast, and Rectal Exams

Occasionally, a patient's complaint will indicate to the candidate that a sensitive examination is required. These exams are prohibited in the COMLEX 2-PE, as noted previously. When candidates think a sensitive exam should be performed, they can advise the patient which exam is recommended and add it to the SOAP note documentation. *Candidates must not actually perform the exam.*

For example, a female patient presents with abdominal pain. The differential diagnosis contains both appendicitis and ovarian cyst. Both a rectal and pelvic examination should be performed. The candidate can simply inform the patient as such:

Candidate: Mrs. Tran, part of your exam should include a pelvic and rectal exam.

The patient will simply refuse. The candidate can thank the patient and move on with discussion of the assessment and plan.

By following the proper technique for examination, candidates for the COMLEX 2-PE can ensure that they receive the highest performance rating during the examination. Candidates should avoid all shortcuts in examination.

REFERENCES

1. National Board of Osteopathic Medical Examiners. *2009–2010 Orientation Guide COMLEX-USA Level 2-PE.* Available at: http://nbome.org/docs/PEOrientationGuide.pdf. Accessed October 9, 2009.

Biomedical/Biomechanical Domain: Assessment and Plan

By now the candidate has completed the history and physical examination and is ready to discuss the findings with the patient. If by the time the 2-minuted warning sounds in the 14-minute encounter the candidate has not completed the history and exam, the candidate *should not* keep examining the patient. A common error made is when candidates try to squeeze in one more exam in the session, and then fail to provide the patient with any diagnosis or plan. The diagnosis and plan are much more important than completing one more part of the neurological exam, for example.

When candidates hear the 2-minute warning, they should finish whichever exam they are currently performing, and then sit down on the stool about 3 to 4 feet from the patient. They should make good eye contact and explain the diagnosis to the patient. The candidate and the patient can then build a plan together. This chapter discusses in more detail these two steps.

ASSESSMENT

The assessment is a list of possible diagnoses, risk factors, or health maintenance issues that candidates develop while working through the standardized patient encounter.

Patients with a Chief Complaint

Candidates should focus on the acute patient concern when a chief complaint is presented.

Primary Diagnoses

If the patient presents with a chief complaint, possible diagnoses will become apparent throughout the history taking. Candidates might add other diagnoses to their list during the problem-specific physical examination. If a diagnosis emerges as a possibility, candidates should note it somewhere on the patient data sheet. As they try to prove their presumptions right or wrong by asking about associated symptoms, candidates can adjust the possible diagnoses based on their likelihood. This is how they develop the differential diagnosis, a list of possible diagnoses with the most likely at the top.

For example, Mr. DiStefano, a 76-year-old man who just returned from wintering in Florida, presents with progressive shortness of breath, cough, and dyspnea on exertion. While obtaining a detailed history using CODIERS SMASH FM, the candidate also finds that the patient has orthopnea, a 10-pound weight gain, and peripheral edema. Considering the possibilities, the candidate proposes heart failure as the most likely diagnosis. The candidate lists this possible diagnosis first; however, she must also consider other possibilities, which might include an acute coronary syndrome resulting in heart failure despite lack of chest pain. During the physical examination, the candidate notes a 2/6 systolic ejection murmur over the aortic valve. She considers severe aortic stenosis, although she would expect a louder murmur, but it is still a possibility. So, the list of possible diagnoses contains heart failure, a possible acute coronary syndrome, and aortic stenosis.

The candidate is entertaining three possible diagnoses from the chief complaint of shortness of breath, cough, and dyspnea on exertion. As a test-taking strategy for the COMLEX 2-PE, candidates must strive for a minimum of four possibilities related to the chief complaint. Three possibilities shows average effort; four or five show diversity of thought and will likely increase the value of their SOAP note. (See Chapter 7, "SOAP Note Documentation.") The diagnoses must be appropriate, however. In the preceding case of Mr. DiStefano, adding pulmonary embolism to the list would be appropriate. On the other hand, aspiration pneumonia is not likely because the patient has no history of vomiting, loss of consciousness, dysphagia, coughing while eating, or alcohol use. The candidate's differential diagnosis now has four primary diagnoses directly related to the chief complaint:

1. Heart failure
2. Possible acute coronary syndrome
3. Aortic stenosis
4. Pulmonary embolism

Documentation of these in order of likelihood is discussed in Chapter 8, "Sample Cases."

Secondary Diagnoses

Secondary diagnoses are the diagnoses the candidate makes that do not relate directly to the chief complaint. For example, a 58-year-old man presents with cough and sputum production. He has a 60-pack per year smoking history. The candidate considers the primary diagnoses to be (1) acute exacerbation of chronic obstructive pulmonary disease (COPD), (2) pneumonia, (3) bronchitis, and (4) lung tumor. All of these are related to the chief complaint. However, while taking his history, the candidate also finds that he drinks 6 beers a day. On his physical examination, the candidate finds a scaly 1-cm lesion on his lower lip. The secondary diagnoses would include (5) alcohol abuse, and (6) a squamous cell carcinoma of the lip. These findings are not directly related to the chief complaint and are, therefore, secondary diagnoses. They do not count toward the extra effort of finding more than three primary diagnoses related to the chief complaint, but they do demonstrate excellent medical care.

1. AECOPD—(Primary diagnosis directly related to Chief Complaint)
2. Pneumonia—(Primary diagnosis directly related to Chief Complaint)
3. Bronchitis—(Primary diagnosis directly related to Chief Complaint)
4. Lung Tumor—(Primary diagnosis directly related to Chief Complaint)
5. Alcohol Abuse—(Secondary Diagnosis)
6. Neoplasm of the Lip—(Secondary Diagnosis)

Be wary, however, of including any diagnosis that does not match the patient encounter. For example, adding to the differential diagnosis acute coronary syndrome for chest pain in a 7-year-old girl just so that there are four diagnoses will likely lead to a lower score because of improper diagnosis than will having only three possibilities listed.

Patients Without a Chief Complaint

Many of the standardized patient encounters lack a true chief complaint. The purpose of these visits is for well visits, health maintenance, or counseling. Examples include annual physical examinations, school or sports physical examinations, or driver's license examinations. Other possibilities include patients who present because family members with specific diagnoses prompted them to come see a physician, for example, the son of a father diagnosed with colorectal cancer presents, or the daughter of a mother with breast cancer, or the sibling of a brother with a heart attack. These patients seek advice and screening for those conditions.

In these cases, candidates need not abandon CODIERS SMASH FM. Although the applicability of CODIERS is certainly limited when there is no chief complaint, candidates can focus strongly on SMASH FM. In these cases, candidates should concentrate on problems that they encounter in the history taking such as excessive alcohol intake, risk factors including a diet high in cholesterol, and smoking in a patient with a family history of stroke or acute coronary syndrome. Health maintenance issues may also present. For example, a patient with a cut—when was his last tetanus booster?

Just as they listed possible diagnoses that arose from the chief complaint, candidates should make a list of the problems, risk factors, and health maintenance issues that they uncover during the history taking and exam.[1p8] They can write these in the SOAP note in the Assessment section.

Sharing the Diagnosis with the Patient

Despite the fact that for the exam candidates will develop an assessment with at least four possible diagnoses related to the chief complaint, candidates need not share each in detail with the patient. When relating a diagnosis to the patient, the candidate should advise the person of the most likely diagnosis,— not all of the possibilities from the differential. For example, candidates would *not* say the following:

> **Candidate:** Ms. Lewis, I believe you have a viral upper respiratory tract infection, but it could be seasonal allergies, a bacterial sinusitis, strep pharyngitis, or even pneumonia.

However, candidates can present the likely diagnosis with brief discussion of other diagnoses if their probability is rather high:

> **Candidate:** Ms. Lewis, I believe you have a viral upper respiratory tract infection, but it could also be seasonal allergies. You don't have findings that would suggest a bacterial infection.

In some cases, candidates might not have a definitive diagnosis. Then, once again, candidates can focus on the most likely possibilities but include in their discussion with the patient the diagnostic workup they will prescribe to make the correct diagnosis. For example, Mrs. Cassano, a 38-year-old woman, presents with epigastric pain. The history does not lead to a finite diagnosis. The discussion of the assessment may go something like this:

> **Candidate:** Mrs. Cassano, I'm not exactly sure what it is that is causing your abdominal pain. There are several different things we should consider. Most of the symptoms you are describing point to your gallbladder; however, there is a possibility that it is your stomach or small intestine, like an ulcer. I'm going to start by getting an ultrasound of your gallbladder and we'll go from there.

THE PLAN

The plan is the culmination of the candidate's thought processes. Diagnoses have been ascertained and a plan of action must be formulated. Although the physician guides the treatment plan, it should be devised with input from the patient, improving their compliance with its implementation.

MOTHRR

At this point, the candidate has provided the patient with the most likely diagnosis. Candidates can then use the mnemonic MOTHRR to prescribe a concise treatment plan. (They should write MOTHRR on the patient data sheet before they enter the patient room.) MOTHRR stands for medications, OMM, testing, holistic/humanistic, referrals, and return visit.

M: Medications

Medications are an obvious place to start because medications are one of the most frequent therapeutic interventions. It is usually easy to think of what to give the patient to treat the patient's symptoms, but candidates must not forget that they must also consider the need to change the dose of or discontinue previously prescribed drugs. Candidates can ask themselves these questions:

- Are there any medications that I can give the patient to treat the primary diagnosis?
  - Example: The candidate diagnoses strep pharyngitis and prescribes Penicillin VK (penicillin with potassium).

- Are there any medications that the patient is taking that may be causing the problem the patient is experiencing, and if so, should I advise the patient to discontinue this medication?
  - Example: A patient with arthritis presents with abdominal pain and is taking 800 mg of ibuprofen 4 times a day. This dose is too high and may be causing the problem, so the candidate adjusts the dose.
- Are there any medications that I should prescribe for the patient for the secondary diagnoses?
  - Example: In the review of the patient's medical history, the candidate finds that the patient has a bee sting allergy. The candidate confirms that the patient has unexpired EpiPens (epinephrine auto injectors) available.

Candidates should advise the patient of any medications that they are adding. It is acceptable to advise the patient on the class of medications if the candidate does not know the exact name during the encounter. (In the clinical setting, physicians have the opportunity to look up the medication and exact dosing and frequency, but this opportunity is not available during the exam.)

> **Candidate:** Mr. Stoner, I am prescribing steroid cream for your rash.

Candidates should provide as much information as they can, which includes medication names, doses, frequencies, directions, and side effects:

> **Candidate:** Mr. Kendall, I want you take a medication called Motrin. It is a nonsteroidal anti-inflammatory, which means that it treats both pain and inflammation. You should take 3 tablets, which is 600 mg, 3 times a day. Take the Motrin with food to help protect your stomach because it can cause some irritation there. If you develop any stomach pain or dark stools, please stop the medication and let me know right away.

O: OMM

After discussing medications with the patient, candidates can next address osteopathic manipulative medicine (OMM). Candidates should consider OMM for every standardized patient encounter; however, by no means should they perform osteopathic manipulation (OM) on every patient because it is not indicated as a standard of care. For example, if a patient presents with acute appendicitis, the candidate should attempt to locate viscerosomatic Chapman points during the physical examination; however, OMM is not indicated. In a pilot study, only 25% of the patient encounters were scored for osteopathic manipulation.[2]

Because of case confidentiality, the exact percentage of cases with expected OMM intervention cannot be ascertained; however, it may be reasonable to hypothesize that OMM is expected for 3 to 5 of the 12 cases candidates encounter on the COMLEX 2-PE. With certainty, OMM should definitely not be "shotgunned" and used for every case because the interpretation will be that the candidate could not ascertain when OMM was truly indicated.

When Is OMM Indicated?

Typically, one of the first questions candidates ask the patient during the history is "When did this start?" Soon thereafter, they should ask the patient whether he or she has ever had this before. If the answer is yes, candidates must follow this lead and ask the patient how the issue resolved. The answer may provide a clue as to whether to apply OMT. For example, when a patient states something like, "Oh, my doctor did something with her hands. It really helped," essentially this says that OMM is expected for the case.

If the candidate determines that OMM is appropriate during the examination, he should ask the patient whether he or she is familiar with osteopathic manipulation. If not, the candidate can briefly describe the philosophy and offer OMM to the patient. Candidates must obtain permission to perform OMM before manipulating any patient.

Obviously, if a patient presents with a musculoskeletal complaint, candidates should include manipulation in the treatment. They must not deem the injury too acute or painful for treatment. There are many techniques that they can use. Candidates must remember that manipulation promotes healing and improves pain. They can use myofascial or muscle energy techniques. They can improve lymphatic drainage to promote circulation and speed healing. Candidates should avoid stating that they would like to bring the patient back for a future visit to perform manipulation. They must perform it during the current encounter unless there are obvious contraindications. Candidates should limit the duration of OMM to 3 to 5 minutes during the encounter.

If you think OMM is indicated ..... then Do it.

OMT Guidelines

Guidelines for manipulation during the examination have been designed by the National Board of Osteopathic Medical Examiners (NBOME) to protect the standardized patients. These guidelines are shown in Table 6–1.[1p7] Table 6–2 shows techniques that are commonly used during standardized patient encounters.[1p7]

Standardized patients undergo manipulation multiple times per day. In consideration of this fact, high velocity low amplitude (HVLA) and techniques where a barrier is engaged and thrust is applied are prohibited.[1p7] Although these techniques are prohibited from use during the examination, if the candidate thinks that they are indicated for the proposed diagnosis, the candidate must document the intent to use them in the written Plan part of the SOAP note.[1p7]

OMM Scoring

Based on the pilot study, scoring for the OMT component consists of 15 measurable components for each case where OMT is expected to be performed. Each of the 15 items could be awarded up to 2 points, for a total of 30 points per OMT encounter. No points are awarded if the measure is skipped or done inappropriately. One point is awarded if the candidate performs the measure correctly, yet hesitates or seems unsure of technique, thereby disrupting fluidity of performance.[2] To obtain maximum points, candidates should demonstrate confidence in their approach.

Some of the 15 areas measured in the pilot study are the following:

- Patient position
- Physician position
- Length of treatment—limit to 5 minutes maximum

Table 6–1 General OMT Guidelines

HVLA techniques are prohibited.
Thrust techniques through an engaged barrier are prohibited.
Gentle techniques must be used at all times.
Limit duration of OMT to under 3 to 5 minutes.
Discontinue the current technique if the patient indicates it is causing any discomfort.
Note: HVLA = high velocity low amplitude.

Table 6–2 Recommended OMT Techniques

Counterstrain
Cranial osteopathy
Facilitated positional release
Galbreath technique
Lymphatic techniques
Muscle energy
Myofascial
Sinus drainage techniques
Still technique
Spencer technique

- Timing of treatment
- Proper hand placement

It is safe to assume that some of these measures continue to represent those evaluated on the COMLEX 2-PE. Other likely areas of measure may include these:

- Appropriate technique for complaint area such as utilization of Spencer technique for shoulder complaints
- Obtaining history of prior osteopathic manipulation

Again, candidates should briefly consider OMM for every patient. However, they must not perform osteopathic treatment for every case. It is likely that 3 to 5 of the 12 cases they encounter during the day of the examination require OMM. Certainly, OMM should be performed for any musculoskeletal complaint, but candidates must also remember to consider it for other diagnoses as well.

T: Testing

Testing includes all of the tests the candidate wants to order to confirm the diagnosis, rule out less likely diagnoses, and guide the treatment plan. This includes such tests as blood work and imaging studies. Candidates should advise the patient about which tests they are ordering, when the patient should have them performed, and when the candidate will advise the patient of the results.

H: Holistic/Humanistic

When relating the plan to the patient, candidates encounter one of the last opportunities to really bond with the patient. Holistically, what can the candidate add to the treatment plan to treat the patient as a whole? If the patient has an infection, can the candidate send him or her back to class or work to contaminate others? How does the patient's current condition affect his or her activities of daily living? Can the patient cook or clean for him- or herself or need help of some sort? Did the candidate provide rest, ice, compression, and elevation (RICE) for injuries?

Humanistically, candidates must ask the patient whether he or she would like them to speak with a relative or friend about the patient's condition. Candidates should get into the habit of asking this question of every patient because it may not seem obvious to do so in certain cases, such as that of a 23-year-old with a sore throat, yet this point is evaluated by the standardized patients. Candidates should take this time to be sure that they have expressed compassion and sympathy and let the patient know that they understand how the condition is affecting him or her. Candidates should let the patient know that the condition and the patient's recovery are important to them.

R: Referrals

Not every case requires a referral. If the candidate deems a referral is appropriate, she should advise the patient of the referral she is making. Candidates must assure the patient that they will communicate with whomever they are referring to and plan for follow-up once the patient has had the referral appointment.

R: Return Visit

Finally, candidates should inform the patient of the follow-up plan. Candidates must not make a referral and then wash their hands of the case. Every case needs a follow-up. How candidates do this is their choice. If a patient comes in with rash for which the candidate prescribes an antihistamine, the candidate can choose to have a nursing staff member call the patient in 2 days to see how the medication is working. A candidate may decide to bring a patient back in to see the nurse for a repeat blood pressure. Or the candidate may need to see a patient again for additional manipulation. Candidates can choose to have a patient come back in 3 weeks, 1 week after a visit with a specialist or following an imaging study, to go over the results. In an encounter where hospitalization is required, admission to the hospital can be considered the follow-up because a true follow-up visit cannot be scheduled until outcomes of the hospitalization have occurred.

The point is, every patient must know and understand when and how follow-up will occur.

EXITING THE ROOM

After candidates have given the patient the diagnosis and built a plan of treatment together, they must be sure to end the encounter with politeness and gratitude. They can ask the patient whether he or she has any questions and sincerely thank patients for their time. Candidates should shake their hand and leave them with a smile.

REFERENCES

1. National Board of Osteopathic Medical Examiners. *2009–2010 Orientation Guide COMLEX-USA Level 2-PE*. Available at: http://nbome.org/docs/PEOrientationGuide.pdf. Accessed October 9, 2009.
2. Gimpel JR, Boulet JR, Errichetti AM. Evaluating the clinical skills of osteopathic medical candidates. *JAOA*. June 2003;103:269-271.

SOAP Note Documentation

CHAPTER

7

Theodore Makoske, MD

At the end of the standardized patient encounter, the candidate has 9 minutes to complete a subjective, objective, assessment, plan (SOAP) note documenting the history obtained, the physical examination performed, the assessment, and plan including any osteopathic manipulative treatment (OMT) that was performed. A SOAP note form that breaks down the areas of documentation into components, as shown in Table 7–1, is given to the candidate for completion.

Further examples of the form utilized during the COMLEX 2-PE and a sample SOAP note can be found on the NBOME website at www.nbome.org.[1pp9–10]

WRITING THE SOAP NOTE

All SOAP notes must be written in the English language. Legibility is also important. Illegible work makes it difficult for the SOAP note evaluator to give proper credit while reviewing the case. **Candidates must not write outside of the boxes**. In addition to appearing sloppy, any writing outside of the boxes is disregarded and does not count toward the SOAP note content.

↱ **Each note must begin with the date and time of the encounter**. This is a medical/legal, coding, and basic good medical practice necessity. A well-written note becomes an accurate account of the patient's current illness followed by the patient's general medical history. This is followed by the findings from the physical examination. The assessment is a list of possible diagnoses that demonstrate the candidate's thought processes and interpretation of the history and exam. Candidates finish the document with what they plan to do for the patient, not only immediately but in the long term as well.

Candidates should avoid using abbreviations in the SOAP note. Although acceptable abbreviations are provided on the NBOME website,[1p11] and Appendix B provides another source for common medical abbreviations[2] as taken from *History and Physical Examination: A Common Sense Approach*, it is very important that candidates avoid using nonstandard abbreviations. It is in the candidate's best interest to avoid using abbreviations all together.

The note should be complete and concise, providing a reader unfamiliar with the case a detailed, easily understood picture of the patient encounter. When practicing with the cases in Chapter 8, candidates can finish each interview by timing themselves as they write a 9-minute SOAP note. They might find that sticking to the 9 minutes is quite a challenge at first.

The standard SOAP note format is shown in Table 7–2.

SUBJECTIVE

The Subjective section of the SOAP note contains only the history that was obtained from the patient encounter. This is the patient's story, collected through using the CODIERS SMASH FM mnemonic tool.

Table 7-1 Blank SOAP Note Form

Subjective

Objective

Assessment

Plan

Table 7–2 SOAP Note Format with Components

Subjective	History only:
	Chief complaint
	CODIERS (in paragraph form)
	SMASH FM (in bulleted format)
Objective	Physical examination:
	System headings
	Osteopathic findings
	Labs
Assessment	Differential diagnosis in order of likelihood
Plan	Therapeutic plan: MOTHRR with notation of intent to perform prohibited or forgotten examinations.

By carefully interviewing the patient, candidates can try to obtain the most thorough and accurate information possible. They may quote the patient directly if the patient uses words or phrases that are not specific diagnoses. Phrases like "fluid on the lungs" or "a cancer in the belly" are acceptable once candidates have done their best to obtain more precise information. By the same token, the patient's ability to recall dates may not be precise. Patients may remember only that they had a tonsillectomy "in childhood" or that they had asthma that "went away in high school," and candidates can record the information as it is presented to them.

The Subjective section always begins with the chief complaint and should be concise, describing the symptoms, diagnosis, or other reasons for the encounter and using the patient's own words as often as practical. The following is an example of how chief complaints should be documented:

> **Subjective 7/21/09 1310**
> **CC: Nasal congestion and frontal headache × 5 days**

After the chief complaint, candidates record the CODIERS portion of the history in paragraph form. This part starts with the patient demographics and gives the patient's age, race, and gender: "19-year-old Caucasian Female complaining of," for example. The rest of the history of the present illness should complete a paragraph giving all of the pertinent information from CODIERS, as in the following example:

> **Subjective 7/21/09 1310**
> **CC: Nasal congestion and frontal Headache × 5 days**
>
> **S: 19-year-old Caucasian Female [demographics] presents c/o nasal congestion with thick green rhinorrhea × 5 days. Also c/o bilateral frontal Headache × 3 days, increased with bending over, postnasal drainage and cough with green sputum production especially in the AM. Rates Headache with a 5/10 intensity. No prior history of the same. Denies sore throat, fever, chills, sob, ear or neck pain.**
> **[paragraph form]**

When candidates first start writing SOAP notes, they may find it difficult to decide exactly which information to include. They can start by following the CODIERS questions very closely, converting the answers to declarative sentences. As they gain skill in creating the narrative of SOAP notes, they should find that they are thinking ahead to the assessment and plan while writing down the subjective material. When they are getting very good at writing a SOAP note, the note should become a cohesive story from start to finish. Once they are able to decide in advance what they want to express in the assessment and plan candidates will have a better idea of what is needed in the Subjective section to support it.

For example, if the candidate thinks that a patient with coughing, sneezing, and a runny nose has a cold, he should carefully describe the symptoms that convinced him of the diagnosis (pertinent positives), and then include all of the factors that helped him decide that the patient did not have other conditions associated with each of those symptoms such as allergies or sinusitis (pertinent negatives).

The SMASH FM information should consist of short lists of information in outline format. Remember that the CODIERS (FED TACOS) SMASH FM mnemonic is a tool for use while learning the art of history taking and for guidance in taking detailed, complete histories. The individual initials do not have any specific meaning in the world of medical documentation, so candidates need to write out the words they stand for or use an accepted abbreviation. Documenting "M: None" is not intelligible to anyone, so candidates should instead write out "Medical History: None."

Once again it is important to include the negative information. The candidate may know that the patient has never been hospitalized, but no one else does until the candidate writes it out. It is also important for candidates to remember to be very specific in asking patients their history to be sure to get the exact information they are seeking. A perfectly compliant patient might tell the candidate that she has no medical conditions, no medications, and no surgeries, and then say that she has been hospitalized five times for pneumonia in the last year—but only if the candidate asks.

Subjective 7/21/09 1310
CC: Nasal congestion and frontal Headache × 5 days

S: 19-year-old Caucasian Female presents c/o nasal congestion with thick green rhinorrhea × 5 days. Also c/o bilateral frontal Headache × 3 days, increased with bending over, postnasal drainage and cough with green sputum production especially in the AM. Rates HA with a 5/10 intensity. No prior history of the same. Denies sore throat, fever, chills, sob, ear or neck pain.

- **Social Hx: Tobacco:** $^1/_2$ ppd × 4 years [SMASH FM bulleted]
- **Alcohol: None**
- **Occupation: College freshman**
- **FDLMP: 1 week ago**
- **Medical Hx: Otitis media—childhood**
- **Allergies: None**
- **Surg Hx: Bilateral ear tubes at 4 y/o**
- **Family Hx: No contacts with similar symptoms**
- **Medications: Birth control pill**

A frequently seen error is putting CODIERS under Subjective and SMASH FM under Objective where the physical examination belongs, and then completely omitting the physical exam from documentation. Candidates should avoid this mistake.

OBJECTIVE

In the Objective section, candidates can begin with transferring the vital signs provided from the patient data sheet. This is the only physical exam documentation that candidates can take from the patient data sheet because everything else they must document from their true findings with the standardized patient. If candidates repeat any vitals, they must mark them as such: "Repeated vitals: BP 132/76 Right arm."

The next lines should contain the physical examination in outline format with headings for each part of the system exam. It is up to the candidate to include as many parts of the physical examination as necessary to give a complete evaluation of the patient's complaint in a concise format while under time pressure. Candidates must remember that this is a problem-specific examination. They can be as detailed and limited as they think is warranted with one possible exception: in almost every case, candidates should include a brief assessment of the heart and lungs. The stethoscope is a symbol of the physician's profession and using it gives the patient an almost subliminal reassurance that the practitioner is doing a "proper" physical examination. Holistically, it could also be argued that unless the heart and lungs are functioning properly, the patient will not be able to heal effectively. Unless the chief complaint is very minor and the patient extremely healthy (a splinter in the finger of a 12-year-old child), candidates should include an assessment of the heart and lungs.

The examination should be written up in the following format:

Objective

Well Developed Well Nourished Caucasian Female in no apparent distress
Temp: 99.0F Pulse: 88 Resp: 16 BP: 160/94 Repeated Blood Pressure: 136/82 R arm Skin: warm and dry without rash
Head: Normocephalic, frontal sinus tenderness to palpation and percussion b/l
Ears: TM's gray b/l with good light reflex
Nose: mucosa edema and erythema with green exudate
Pharynx: minimal erythema, green Post-nasal drainage. No tonsillar hypertrophy.
Neck: without lymphadenopathy
Lungs: Clear to auscultation without wheezes, crackles
Heart: Regular Rhythm without murmur, rub, or gallop

In an ideal physical examination, candidates would include every positive finding that helps to confirm the most likely diagnosis and any negative finding that help to exclude other items in the differential. If, while working on the write-up, the candidate decides that a part of the examination is not meaningful to the current complaint, she is not obligated to record it. If the candidate checked pupillary response while examining a patient with an upper respiratory infection, there is no reason why the candidate has to take time to write it down if it has nothing to do with the final diagnosis. **Candidates must, however, be very careful not to write anything in the physical exam that they did not actually do.** They are allowed to state things they intend to do in the future in the Plan section, but the Objective area is restricted to current factual information. Any statements in this part of the note that cannot be confirmed by the standardized patient or by reviewing the candidate's video record are considered irregular behavior and could result in the entire test being disqualified, resulting in failure of the examination.

ASSESSMENT

The assessment is the differential diagnosis and should be numbered in order of likelihood. **Again, as a test-taking strategy, candidates need to include a minimum of four possible diagnoses that relate directly to the chief complaint.** Typically, the differential is very straightforward. For the patient with coughing, sneezing, and runny nose, candidates could simply write the following:

Assessment
1. Sinusitis
2. Rhinitis
3. URI
4. Doubt seasonal allergies

Though the diagnoses do not have to match the patient's presentation perfectly, they must address part of the chief complaint. In some cases, the first item listed may be the most obvious diagnosis possible and the others may be more unlikely, but listing four diagnoses not only displays candidates' medical knowledge, it also shows that candidates did not develop tunnel vision and ignore other possible causes of the patient's condition.

It is permissible to start the additional diagnoses with the phrase "*Rule out*" if the candidate thinks that they are possible but would require further testing to be certain. With the most likely diagnoses listed first, the candidate can put the word *doubt* in front of the additional items to show that even though he considered them, they are least likely based on his findings. **It is important for candidates to remember that their first item in the differential diagnosis should be the most likely choice and must always be a positive statement, not something they "doubt" or want to "rule out."**

If there is no actual complaint in the reason for the patient's visit, such as when a patient presents for a routine physical exam, candidates should list preexisting medical problems, health maintenance issues, or risk factors appropriate to the patient's age.[1p8] For example, a 50-year-old diabetic man presents for a yearly physical examination, which is required for him to drive a school bus. He smokes, has an allergy to bee stings, and is noted to have a mild elevation of his blood pressure with no history of prior elevation. The assessment might include items such as follows:

Assessment
1. **Diabetes mellitus** [preexisting medical condition]
2. **Tobacco use disorder** [risk factor]
3. **Elevated Blood Pressure without diagnosis of hypertension** [risk factor]
4. **Bee sting allergy** [preexisting condition]
5. **Colorectal cancer screening** [health maintenance issue]

Assessment Scoring

In documentation of the assessment, three diagnoses directly related to the chief complaint is considered an average effort. As long as the diagnoses are appropriate for the differential, candidates would do well to expand the differential. They can do this by giving one or two more diagnoses directly based on the chief complaint.

It is very important that any diagnosis the candidate entertains for the differential be supported by the history and physical examination. For example, if a patient presents with dark, tarry stools and has epigastric pain on palpation, including *lung tumor* in the differential has no basis and would affect the scoring of the encounter adversely. **Likewise, if the candidate lists somatic dysfunction as one of the differentials, somewhere in the physical examination there must be documentation of the dysfunction such as a palpatory finding, restriction, or detected viscerosomatic reflex**.

Secondary diagnoses not related to the chief complaint should also be noted lower on the differential. Candidates can include such items as tobacco abuse disorder, excess alcohol consumption, or any other medical problem that the patient may have that is not directly related to the reason for the patient's visit. They can include health maintenance issues or risk factors, for example, a 50-year-old patient presenting for a routine physical. Candidates should advise him of the need for a rectal exam and colorectal cancer screening.

PLAN

After being very thorough and demonstrating their medical knowledge by expanding the differential diagnoses to more than three possibilities in the Assessment portion of the note, candidates must shift gears when it comes to the plan. The first priority in the Plan section is to give a well-thought-out course of treatment for the diagnosis the candidate thinks is most likely and to include as many elements of proper medical care as possible. Candidates may also rule out secondary diagnoses as appropriate. For example, in a patient with a likely urinary tract infection (URI), the candidate can address and rule out strep pharyngitis effectively with a simple notation of "throat culture" in the plan.

MOTHRR

By using the mnemonic MOTHRR, candidates can cover all of the elements needed to construct a complete plan for the patient. As discussed in Chapter 6, MOTHRR stands for:

- Medicines
- Osteopathic treatment
- Testing
- Holistic/humanistic items
- Referrals
- Return visit

Not every aspect of this mnemonic is required for every case, but candidates should at least think of each category as they decide on the appropriate treatment for patients. Candidates must also remember that the letters used in the mnemonic are meaningless to anyone other than them. They can either write out the individual headings or simply number the items that address each of the categories—they must not simply write out the letters M-O-T-H-R-R as headings.

Medications

The COMLEX 2-PE does not require candidates to specify particular drug doses or names, but candidates should be as precise as possible in stating the course of treatment. They must document the drug name, dose, and frequency if possible, and give broad categories if they are unable to give specifics. For example, "NSAIDS" is acceptable; however, "ibuprofen 600 mg PO 3 times a day with food" is better.

Osteopathic Manipulative Medicine

To offer and perform osteopathic manipulative medicine (OMM) on a patient, candidates must be certain to include in the differential the dysfunction necessitating manipulation. Performing OMM without an associated diagnosis is inappropriate.

Once the candidate has a diagnosis, has determined OMM is appropriate, and has performed it, he must document it, noting areas of treatment and techniques used. If the candidate gets to this portion of the Plan section and realizes that there was a treatment he could have performed but did not, he cannot say that he did. In addition, because no high velocity low amplitude (HVLA) is allowed on standardized patients, if the candidate thinks that HVLA is appropriate, he should note it here in the plan.[1p7] Documenting that OMM was performed in the SOAP while not actually doing it would be labeled as irregular, again resulting in failure. If this is the case, candidates should write in the Plan section that it should have been offered and recommend it being done at the patient follow-up.

Testing

Testing includes all of the tests the candidate wants to order to confirm the diagnosis, rule out less likely diagnoses, and guide the treatment plan. This includes such items as blood work, radiological studies, and specialized tests performed by other providers. In this section, avoid laboratory panels that vary from testing site to testing site such as "Chem 14." Candidates should be as specific as possible and order specific tests such as BUN, creatinine, and glucose. Candidates display their medical knowledge to greater advantage by asking for specific tests rather than by using a shotgun approach to cover all the possibilities.

Holistic/Humanistic

Holistic/humanistic items show the candidate's concern for the patient as a whole and demonstrate that the candidate is thinking of the patient as a person rather than as a simple diagnosis. **Classic examples of displaying holistic and humanistic care is when the candidate asks whether the patient would like her to speak with a relative or friend about the patient's condition and when the candidate asks questions that indicate that she is thinking about how the current illness is affecting the patient's life by interfering with work or activities of daily living.** Candidates should ask these types of questions of every patient because they are very likely evaluated by the standardized patient. By writing in their plan that they are going to take steps to overcome these problems, candidates give concrete evidence that they have considered these matters carefully.

Referral

Referral is another area where candidates will not always have something to add. If a candidate is convinced that he needs the help of a specialist to take care of the patient, then by all means he should ask for one. But candidates should not order excessive consultations simply to have something to put in this category. Candidates must also remember that as fully trained osteopathic physicians, they are competent to take care of most medical conditions that present in the environment of a primary care or ambulatory clinic setting, which the COMLEX 2-PE is meant to reflect. If the setting is an emergency room, more referrals are expected, such as surgery for appendicitis or orthopedics for a fracture. However, candidates do not need an orthopedic surgeon for every sprained ankle, and they can handle simple diabetes without an endocrinologist.

Return Visit

The return visit is the last thing to address. If the candidate is going to admit the patient to the hospital, then she does not need to have a return plan until it is time to discharge the patient. In all other instances, candidates should indicate that they plan to see this patient again. As dedicated physicians who are committed to the idea of making certain that their patients are completely recovered from illness, candidates need to follow up with the patients. They cannot rest until they have done everything in their power to return individuals to an optimal state of homeostasis, and candidates show this by always scheduling a return visit, follow-up phone call, or some other interaction to provide completeness to the encounter.

If candidates are uncertain about the correct interval until the next visit, they should err on the side of sooner rather than later. Bringing patients back to the office in 1 week shows concern for their well-being.

Plan
Medications: Amoxicillin 500 mg tid × 14 days
OMM: Frontal sinus drainage techniques applied b/l
Holistic: Increase fluids, return to work in 2 days
Return visit: Nursing to call in 3 days to reassess. Patient to call earlier with increase in headache, fever, change in vision, no improvement.

FALSE DOCUMENTATION

A candidate should *never* document any history that was not actually asked or document portions of the examination or osteopathic manipulation that were not truly performed. If, after leaving the examination room and writing the SOAP note, the candidate realizes that he forgot to obtain certain information or perform particular examinations, he should write in the SOAP note his intent to return to the patient and do so. Video recordings are made of each standardized patient encounter and are compared to the SOAP note. False documentation is aggressively investigated, as described in the NBOME's *Bulletin of Information*.[1p12,3p28] If the candidate documents history that he did not ask or exams and manipulation that he did not perform, because this is deemed a violation of professionalism competency, his test will be marked as "irregular" and thrown out, resulting in failure of the examination. This means the candidate will have to retake the examination and pay the examination fees again.[1p8]

STOP WRITING!

A 2-minute warning is given to alert candidates that the 9-minute SOAP note documentation session is nearing an end. Candidates should be prepared to stop writing immediately when the 9 minutes has elapsed. **When the session end is announced, candidates must *stop writing*!** If they do not,

Table 7-3 Complete SOAP Note Documentation Sample

Subjective 7/21/09 1310

CC: Nasal congestion and frontal Headache × 5 days

S: 19-year old Caucasian female presents c/o nasal congestion with thick green rhinorrhea ¥ 5 days. Also c/o bilateral frontal Headache × 3 days, increased with bending over, postnasal drainage and cough with green sputum production especially in the AM. Rates Headache with a 5/10 intensity. No prior history of the same. Denies sore throat, fever, chills, sob, ear or neck pain.

Social Hx: Tobacco: $^1/_2$ ppd × 4 years

Alcohol: None

Occupation: College freshman

FDLMP: 1 week ago

Medical Hx: Otitis media—childhood

Allergies: None

Surg Hx: Bilateral ear tubes at 4 y/o

Family Hx: No contacts with similar symptoms

Medications: Birth control pill

Objective

Well Developed Well Nourished Caucasian Female in no apparent distress

Temp: 99.0F   Pulse: 88   Resp: 16   Blood pressure: 160/94   Repeated BP: 136/82 Right arm

Skin: Warm and dry without rash

Head: Normocephalic, frontal sinus tenderness to palpation and percussion b/l

Ears: TM's gray b/l with good light reflex

Nose: Mucosa edema and erythema with green exudate

Pharynx: Minimal erythema, green Post-nasal drainage. No tonsillar hypertrophy.

Neck: without lymphadenopathy

Lungs: Clear to auscultation without wheezes, crackles

Heart: Regular rhythm w/o murmur, rub, or gallop

Assessment

1. Assessment
2. Sinusitis
3. URI
4. Doubt seasonal allergies
5. Tobacco use disorder

Plan

Medications: Amoxicillin 500 mg tid × 14 days

OMM: Frontal sinus drainage techniques applied b/l

Holistic: Increase fluids, return to work in 2 days

Return plan: Nursing to call in 3 days to reassess. Patient to call earlier with increase in headache, fever, change in vision, no improvement.

they will receive a warning. If it occurs again, they will fail the exam, pure and simple.[3p29] Candidates must not try to finish the sentence they are on. They just must stop. An incomplete note carries much less penalty than that of an overall failure. While doing the cases in Chapter 8, candidates should practice writing the notes in 9 minutes. Some candidates opt to document the Assessment and Plan first, and then the Subjective and Objective sections.

SOAP NOTE SCORING

Based on the pilot study data, scoring of SOAP note documentation of the encounter is derived by grading each section, Subjective, Objective, Assessment, and Plan, of the SOAP note and one overall score. The grading range is from 1 to 9 with 9 being the highest possible grade obtainable. An additional overall performance score is given for accuracy, synthesis of the data, structure, and legibility.[4]

REFERENCES

1. National Board of Osteopathic Medical Examiners. *2009–2010 Orientation Guide COMLEX-USA Level 2-PE*. Available at: http://nbome.org/docs/PEOrientationGuide.pdf. Accessed October 9, 2009.
2. Kauffman M, Roth-Kauffman M. *The History and Physical Examination Workbook: A Common Sense Approach*. Boston: Jones and Bartlett; 2007.
3. National Board of Osteopathic Medical Examiners. *Bulletin of Information 2009–2010*. Available at: http://nbome.org/docs/comlexBOI.pdf. Accessed October 11, 2009.
4. Gimpel JR, Boulet JR, Errichetti AM. Evaluating the clinical skills of osteopathic medical candidates. *JAOA*. June 2003;103:269-271.

Sample Cases

Michele M. Roth-Kauffman, JD, MPAS, PA-C

CHAPTER

8

WHAT TO EXPECT ON THE COMLEX 2-PE

Case development by the National Board of Osteopathic Medical Examiners (NBOME) is reportedly based on chief complaints commonly encountered in osteopathic primary care settings.[1p7] The cases are designed to lead to particular diagnostic outcomes.[2] In addition, the clinical cases represent a wide array of patient age, sex, and race demographics reflecting a typical outpatient primary care population and are based on the National Ambulatory Medical Care Survey Data.[3]

Patient encounters with their chief complaints may be acute such as injuries or infectious disease concerns, or chronic in nature such as patients presenting for follow-up on hypertension or diabetes. These cases are broken down into categories of symptoms, each comprising a percentage of the cases that candidates may encounter. These clinical presentations follow the "Dimension I Blueprint" of the COMLEX Levels 1, 2, and 3 and are designed to identify the most commonly seen clinical scenarios or reflect health issues that are considered "high impact."[1p14]

Candidates should anticipate cases lacking chief complaints and cases that may focus on preventative health care such as child, adolescent, and adult well visits where patient age would dictate appropriate education and instruction, such as recommending colorectal cancer screening at well adult visits when patients are nearing 50 years of age. Candidates can also expect to encounter birth control issues and obstetrical-related cases as they would in true clinical settings.

Detailed topics covered by each category are in the CBT Tutorial available on the NBOME website (www.nbome.org).

Clinical presentations derived from the Dimension I Blueprint identify the following areas for case development[1p17]:

- Digestion
- Metabolism
- Neurosensory
- Neuromuscular
- Genitourinary
- Human sexuality
- Respiratory
- Circulatory
- Thermoregulation
- Integumentary
- Trauma
- Human development
- Generalized or asymptomatic presentations

65

The *Bulletin of Information* summarizes these areas into the following categories for case development[1p17]:

- Patients with Neuromusculoskeletal Symptoms/Problems
- Patients with Respiratory Symptoms/Problems
- Patients with Gastrointestinal Symptoms/Problems
- Patients with Cardiovascular Symptoms/Problems
- Patients with Other Symptoms/Problems

ANTICIPATED CASES

As stated earlier, the Candidate Confidentiality Agreement prohibits any candidate from sharing information about the COMLEX 2-PE after taking the examination. Respecting this position of the NBOME, this author made no attempt to obtain specific content of case samples from prior candidates. However, with literature searches of publications related to the development of this evaluation tool and publicly available descriptions of the COMLEX 2-PE available from the NBOME, this author was able to surmise likely case topics and develop case-based scenarios that likely mimic those that candidates can expect to encounter during the practical examination.

The pilot study of the COMLEX 2-PE from "Evaluating the Clinical Skills of Osteopathic Medical Students," published in the *Journal of American Osteopathic Association* in June 2003, shows that the following cases were encountered[2]:

- Low back pain
- Acute chest pain
- Chronic abdominal pain
- Insomnia/depression
- Infant with gastrointestinal reflux
- Frozen shoulder
- Joint pain/fatigue
- Asthmatic with cough
- Acute dyspnea
- Elderly patient with confusion
- Shortness of breath/chest pain

It is likely that some of these case scenarios are still in use for the examination.

HOW TO UTILIZE THE PRACTICE CASES

Finally, candidates are ready to start practicing patient encounters in the exact format utilized during the COMLEX 2-PE. At this point, they must now bring together history taking and the physical examination. Candidates who take excellent histories and who perform detailed physical examinations may find it quite difficult to bring the two together under the constraints of a 14-minute exercise.

The cases provided are designed as partnered practical examination practice encounters; however, candidates can study the case content individually as well. While one candidate performs the history and physical, the other person is the patient. The candidate who acts as the patient should review the answers to the history questions to become familiar with the scenario. Practice partners may choose to perform the first several cases without a time limit; however, after these first cases, they should progress to the time limits set forth later.

Each case starts with the candidate reviewing the patient data sheet. The patient data sheet contains the patient's name, clinical setting, and chief complaint. It also provides the vital signs. This simulates office settings were triage is performed by other staff members. It is very important for candidates to review the vital signs and repeat them if needed during the examination. For example, if the patient data sheet shows a blood pressure of 140/85 in a diabetic, it would be important for the candidate to repeat the blood pressure because the goal for blood pressure in diabetics is less than 130/80.

Table 8–1 Practice Case Summary

1. Patient reads case history answers.
2. Fourteen-minute timer is started.
3. Candidate reviews patient data sheet.
4. Candidate writes mnemonics on patient data sheet or other paper.
5. Candidate knocks and enters room, making immediate eye contact.
6. Candidate excuses self and washes hands for 15 seconds, turning off water with towel.
7. Candidate shakes patient's hand.
8. Candidate takes history thorough CODIERS SMASH FM and FED TACOS.
9. Candidate performs problem-specific examination.
10. Candidate offers diagnosis.
11. Candidate together with patient develop the treatment plan and candidate offers and performs OMM if appropriate.
12. Candidate asks patient if there are any questions and thanks patient.
13. Candidate leaves the room.
14. Timer reset for 9 minutes plus any additional minutes left over from the 14 minutes allotted for encounter.
15. Candidate documents encounter in a SOAP note.
16. Candidate immediately stops writing at 9 minutes.
17. Candidate reviews the case and the Humanistic domain evaluation.

Practice sessions should mimic the encounter precisely. Table 8–1 provides a summary of steps candidates can use while practicing these encounters, and the process is reviewed in the following paragraphs.

The candidate should stand outside the patient's room, start the timer, and then review the face sheet. Time is not allotted on the exam specifically for reviewing the sheet but is included in the 14 minutes candidates are given. Candidates should write down the mnemonics they will use. Next, they enter the room, make eye contact, wash their hands while taking the opportunity to bond "non-medically" with the patient, and then shake hands and get down to the business of the history taking.

During the 14 minutes, candidates must elicit a history and perform the problem-specific physical examination. These time limits are meant to reflect a typical outpatient visit. If candidates have not started to share the proposed diagnosis with the patient at the 2-minute warning, they should stop what they are doing and do so. Candidates should develop a plan with the patient. Finally, the candidate should ask whether the patient has any questions and thank the patient for the visit. If the end of session is announced, before the candidate has finished, the candidate should thank the patient and immediately leave the room.

While practicing, candidates should not take a break—simply reset the timer for 9 minutes and begin writing a SOAP note on the form provided with each case. Candidates should include at least four possibilities in the differential diagnosis, ranking them in order of likelihood. If no chief complaint was given, candidates can address preventative measures as indicated.

While the candidate writes the SOAP note, the patient should complete the humanistic evaluation, being brutally honest about how he or she felt as a patient.

Candidates should practice these cases until they develop fluidity and precision in the patient encounter while adhering to the 14- and 9-minute time frames. At first, candidates can expect not to complete the encounters within the allotted time. They can identify areas that require the majority of their time and work on improving skills in those areas.

Sample SOAP notes are provided for the first two case encounters. Candidates should practice writing SOAP notes for these cases and compare them to the samples provided. That format should be followed for the remaining cases.

Finally, although many more questions could be asked for each case and additional components of the physical exams can be performed, the cases are designed to provide answers to candidate questions and areas of examination that are deemed to be of high-yield.

REFERENCES

1. National Board of Osteopathic Medical Examiners. *Bulletin of Information 2009–2010*. Available at: http://nbome.org/docs/comlexBOI.pdf. Accessed October 14, 2009.
2. Gimpel, JR, Boulet JR, Errichetti AM. Evaluating the clinical skills of osteopathic medical candidates. *JAOA*. June 2003;103:269–270.
3. Boulet JR, Gimpel JR, Errichetti AM, Meoli FG. Using national medical care survey data to validate examination content on a performance-based clinical skills assessment for osteopathic physicians. *JAOA*. May 2003;103:225.

Case 1

Patient Name: Rita Rieno
Clinical Setting: Family Practice Office
CC: An 18 y/o female presents for "a runny nose."

Vital Signs
Blood pressure: 110/60
Respirations: 14 per minute
Temperature: 98.2°F
Pulse: 68 bpm
Weight: 168 lbs
Height: 5'11"

NOTES:

Subjective

Objective

Assessment

Plan

CC: An 18 y/o female presents for "a runny nose."

History			✓
	1	Introduces self and explains role of provider.	
	2	Properly washes hands before touching the patient (15-sec wash and turns off with towel).	
	3	Opening question: What brings you in today?	My nose won't quit running.	✓
Chronology/ Onset	4	**When** did this start?	It's been the last couple of years, but has gotten really bad the last month.	✓
	5	Did you ever have this **before**?	It never really goes away completely.	
Description	6	Could you **describe the nasal discharge?**	It's clear.	
Exacerbation	7	Does anything make it **worse**?	It's worse in the spring and fall.	
Remission	8	What makes it **better**?	Benadryl helps, but it makes me drowsy.	✓
	9	How **often** do you take Benadryl?	A couple times a week.	✓
	10	How **many milligrams**?	I take 2 tablets. I don't know milligrams.	✓
Symptoms associated	11	Do you have **itchy, watery eyes**?	Yes.	✓
	12	**Headache?**	No.	
	13	**Nasal congestion**?	Yes. Quite a bit.	✓
	14	**Ear pain**?	No.	✓
	15	**Fever**?	No.	
	16	**Sore throat**?	Just scratchy.	✓
	17	**Cough**?	No.	✓
Social Hx	18	Do you **smoke**?	A little.	✓
(FED TACOS)	19	**How much** is "a little"?	A pack lasts me 2 or 3 days.	✓
	20	**How long** have you been smoking?	About a year or two.	✓
	21	Do you drink **alcohol**?	No.	✓
	22	Do you use any **drugs**?	No.	
	23	What is your **occupation**?	I'm a senior in high school.	
Medical Hx	24	Do you have any medical conditions?	No.	✓
Allergies	25	Do you have any allergies?	Cats seem to bother me.	✓
	26	What happens when you are around cats?	My eyes itch and my throat gets scratchy.	✓
Surg Hx	27	Have you had any surgeries?	No.	✓
Hosp Hx	28	Have you ever been hospitalized?	No.	
Family Hx	29	Medical conditions that run in the family?	Yes.	✓
	30	Who?	My father. He has allergies.	✓
Menstrual Hx	31	When was the **FDLMP**?	About a week ago.	✓
Medications	32	Are you on any medications?	Just Benadryl when I need it.	✓

Physical Examination ✓

			✓
	33 Informs patient that the physical exam is to begin and asks permission.		✓
	34 Rewashes hand before touching patient if candidate has recontaminated them.		
Sinuses	35 Palpation	**Mild maxillary sinus tenderness**	✓
Eyes	36 Inspection	**Dark circles are noted under the eyes No periorbital edema noted**	
Ears	37 External inspection	**No exudate**	✓
	38 Otoscopic examination	**TM's gray b/l**	✓
	39 Inverted otoscope with finger distended		
	40 Proper ear position—Adult: up, back, out.		
Nose	41 Inspection with light source	**Boggy turbinates/clear nasal discharge**	✓
Throat	42 Inspection with light source and tongue blade	**Clear postnasal drip present**	✓
Lymphatics	43 Palpation of cervical nodes	**No cervical adenopathy**	✓
Respiratory	44 Auscultation performed on bare skin	**Clear to auscultation**	✓
	45 Through complete inspiration and expiration		
	46 Symmetrically		
	47 At least 2 anterior levels, 1 lateral, and 3 posterior		
Cardiac	48 Auscultation performed on bare skin	**RR without murmurs, rubs, or gallops**	✓
	49 Areas: aortic, pulmonic, tricuspid, and mitral		
Assessment	50 Presents patient with a proposed diagnosis (environmental allergies).		
Plan	51 MTHR: Antihistamine, allergy testing, holistic, smoking cessation, contact avoidance.		
(MOTHRR)	52 Explains and offers OMM.		✓
	53 Performs OMM appropriately (no HVLA).		✓
	54 Return plan: Devises and explains a follow-up plan with the patient.		✓
	55 Thanks the patient and asks if there are any questions.		✓

Humanistic Evaluation Y/N

	Y/N
Did the candidate present in a self-caring manner (e.g., hair control, clothing, cleanliness, aroma, etc.)?	
Did the candidate make periodic eye contact?	
Was the candidate's language clear and EASY to understand?	
Did the candidate have any substance in his or her mouth during the session?	
Did the candidate exhibit body language that would make you feel the candidate was communicating with you?	
Was the candidate enthusiastic?	
Did the candidate exhibit pride in his or her efforts?	
Did the candidate make any comment regarding your lifestyle (e.g., your work, family, activities, etc.)?	
Did the candidate express any humanistic statement recognizing your concerns?	
Did the candidate explain the medical problem and offer you a possible diagnosis?	
Did the candidate suggest a treatment plan that you could understand?	
Did the candidate inquire whether you might want to consult with family members or others about your visit?	
Did the candidate present as if he or she were a competent interviewer?	
Did the candidate ask you if you had any questions?	
Did the candidate thank you?	

Sample SOAP Note Provided for Case 1

Subjective   8/11/2009   0930

CC: Runny Nose

Miss Rieno, an 18 y/o Caucasian female presents with a clear, continuous runny nose that has occurred for the last several years, but that has worsened over the last month. She states the discharge is worse in the spring and fall, but "really never goes away." She has attempted relief with Benadryl a couple times a week, taking two tablets of unknown milligrams with some relief, but admits associated drowsiness. She admits itchy, watery eyes; nasal congestion; and a scratchy throat. She denies cephalgia, ear pain, fever, or cough.

Social History: Tobacco: - 1/2 ppd × 2–3 years   Family History: Father with history
                Alcohol: denies   of allergies
                Drugs: denies   FDLMP - 1 week ago
                Occupation: student   Medications: Benadryl prn as above

Medical history: None

Allergies: environmental—cats

Surgeries: none

Hospitalizations: none

Objective

Vitals: BP 110/60, Resp 14, Pulse 68 bpm, Temp 98.2, Wt 168 lb, Ht 5'11"

General: WDWN in NAD

HEENT: Sinuses: mild maxillary tenderness b/l
        Eyes: infraorbital venous pooling. No periorbital edema
        Ears: TM's gray b/l with good light reflex
        Nose: mucosa pale with boggy turbinates and clear exudate
        Throat: mild clear postnasal drainage

Neck: No lymphadenopathy

Lungs: Clear to auscultation

Heart: Reg rhythm without murmur, rub, or gallop

Assessment

1) Allergic rhinitis
2) Doubt viral rhinosinusitis
3) Doubt bacterial rhinosinusitis
4) Tobacco use disorder exacerbating rhinitis

Plan

1) Histamine antagonist—Cetirizine 5 mg PO daily
2) OMM—sinus drainage technique applied
3) Consider allergy testing. Contact avoidance counseling
4) Provided smoking cessation counseling and offered cessation assistance
5) Return to office in 2 weeks

                                              Lyncean Ung OMS-IV

Case 2

Patient Name:	Harmon Hertz
Clinical Setting:	Family Practice Office
CC:	A 45 y/o male presents for "shoulder pain."

Vital Signs

Blood pressure:	118/75
Respirations:	14 per minute
Temperature:	98°F
Pulse:	88 bpm
Weight:	175 lbs
Height:	5'11"

NOTES:

Subjective

Objective

Assessment

Plan

CC: A 45 y/o male presents for "shoulder pain."

History				✓
	1	Introduces self and explains role of provider.		✓
	2	Properly washes hands before touching the patient (15-sec wash and turns off with towel).		✓
	3	Opening question: What brings you in today?	My left shoulder really hurts.	✓
Chronology/ Onset	4	**When** did this start?	About 2 months ago.	✓
	5	Did you ever have this **before**?	No.	✓
	6	What are you **doing** when it happens?	It started after I painted my house.	✓
	7	Did it come on **suddenly or gradually**?	Gradually.	
Description	8	Could you **describe it**?	It's achy and stiff.	✓
	9	**Where** is it located?	On the outside of my left shoulder.	✓
	10	Does it **radiate/go** anywhere?	No.	
Duration	11	**Does it come and go** or is it **continuous**?	It hurts all the time.	
Intensity	12	How severe is it, on a scale from **1 to 10**?	A 6.	✓
Exacerbation	13	Does anything make it **worse**?	When I try to raise my arm, it's worse.	✓
Remission	14	What makes it **better**?	Keeping still and aspirin.	✓
	15	**How much** aspirin do you take?	650 milligrams	✓
	16	**How often** do you take it?	Two or three times a day.	✓
Symptoms associated	17	**Fever or chills**?	No.	✓
	18	**Other joint pain**?	No.	✓
	19	**Weakness**?	I just can't lift it because of the pain.	✓
	20	**Numbness or tingling**?	No.	✓
	21	**Chest pain**?	No.	✓
	22	**Shortness of breath**?	No.	✓
	23	**Cough**?	No.	✓
Social Hx	24	What does your **diet** look like?	I watch the sweets.	
(FED TACOS)	25	Do you **exercise** using your arm?	Not really. Just with my job.	
	26	Do you use any **drugs**?	No.	✓
	27	Do you use **tobacco**?	No.	✓
	28	Do you drink **alcohol**?	Yes.	✓
	29	**How much** a day?	Just a couple beers a week.	✓
	30	Do you drink **caffeine**?	Two cups of coffee in the morning.	✓
	31	What is your **occupation**?	I deliver newspapers.	
Medical Hx	32	Do you have any medical conditions?	A touch of diabetes.	✓
Allergies	33	Do you have any allergies?	No.	✓
Surg Hx	34	Have you had any surgeries?	No.	✓
Hosp Hx	35	Have you ever been hospitalized?	No.	✓
Family Hx	36	Medical conditions that run in the family?	Diabetes runs in the family.	✓
Medications	37	Are you on any medications?	No. My diabetes is controlled by diet.	✓

Physical Examination ✓

			✓
	38	Informs patient that the physical exam is to begin and asks permission.	✓
	39	Rewashes hands before touching patient if candidate has recontaminated them.	✓
Neck	40	Inspection	**Symmetrical**	
	41	Active range of motion	**Full AROM**	
	42	Palpation	**Nontender to palpation**	
Respiratory	43	Auscultation performed on bare skin	**Clear to auscultation**	✓
	44	Through complete inspiration and expiration		✓
	45	Symmetrically		✓
	46	At least 2 anterior levels, 1 lateral, and 3 posterior		✓
Cardiac	47	Auscultation performed on bare skin	**RR without murmurs, rubs, gallops**	✓
	48	Areas: aortic, pulmonic, tricuspid, and mitral		✓
MS	49	Inspection of bilateral shoulders	**No erythema, ecchymosis, deformity**	
	50	Active ROM b/l shoulders, elbows	**L shoulder limited to 90 degrees abd**	
	51	Passive range of motion for limited R shoulder	**L shoulder is limited to 90 degrees**	
	52	Palpation of bilateral shoulders	**No point tenderness**	
Vascular	53	Brachial and radial pulses compared bilaterally	**2/4 b/l**	
Neurologic	54	Motor: Strength testing with b/l comparison	**Patient hesitant secondary to pain**	
	55	Sensory to sharp/dull, light touch	**Intact**	
	56	Reflexes—b/l upper extremity	**2/4 bicep, triceps, brachioradialis**	
Special Testing	57	Arm drop test	**Negative**	
Assessment	58	Presents patient with a proposed diagnosis.	**Adhesive capsulitis, r/o rotator cuff inj**	
Plan	59	MTHR: Pain control, shoulder X-ray, holistic (RICE), referral		
(MOTHRR)	60	Explains and offers OMM.		✓
	61	Performs OMM appropriately (no HVLA).		✓
	62	Return plan: Devises and explains a follow-up plan with the patient.		
	63	Thanks the patient and asks if there are any questions.		

Humanistic Evaluation Y/N

	Y/N
Did the candidate present in a self-caring manner (e.g., hair control, clothing, cleanliness, aroma, etc.)?	
Did the candidate make periodic eye contact?	
Was the candidate's language clear and EASY to understand?	
Did the candidate have any substance in his or her mouth during the session?	
Did the candidate exhibit body language that would make you feel the candidate was communicating with you?	
Was the candidate enthusiastic?	
Did the candidate exhibit pride in his or her efforts?	
Did the candidate make any comment regarding your lifestyle (e.g., your work, family, activities, etc.)?	
Did the candidate express any humanistic statement recognizing your concerns?	
Did the candidate explain the medical problem and offer you a possible diagnosis?	
Did the candidate suggest a treatment plan that you could understand?	
Did the candidate inquire whether you might want to consult with family members or others about your visit?	
Did the candidate present as if he or she were a competent interviewer?	
Did the candidate ask you if you had any questions?	
Did the candidate thank you?	

Sample SOAP Note Provided for Case 2

Subjective   8/22/2009   1450

CC: Left shoulder pain × 2 months

Mr. Hurtz, a 45 y/o male, presents with left should pain that began 2 months ago shortly after painting his house. No prior episodes of the same. Pain began gradually and is described as "achy and stiff." Patient locates pain on the outside of the left shoulder without radiation. It is continuous and is scaled at 6/10. Attempting to raise his arm makes the pain worse. He gets some relief with keeping the arm still and aspirin 650 mg 2 or 3 times a day. He denies fever, chills, weakness, numbness, tingling, chest pain, shortness of breath, or cough.

Social History:		
	Diet: avoids sweets	Med history: diabetes—dietary control
	Exercise: no regular routine	Allergies: none
	Drugs: denies	Surgeries: none
	Tobacco: denies	Hospitalizations: none
	Alcohol: 2–3 beers per week	Family History: Diabetes
	Caffeine: 2 cups of coffee a day	Medications: Aspirin as above
	Occupation: newspaper delivery	

Objective

Vitals: BP 118/75, Resp 14, Pulse 88 bpm, Temp 98, Wt 175 lb, Ht 5' 11"

General: WDWN in NAD

Neck:	Symmetrical, full active range of motion, nontender to palpation
Lungs:	Clear to auscultation
Heart:	Reg rhythm without murmur, rub, or gallop
MS:	Bilateral shoulders without erythema, ecchymosis, or deformity. Right shoulder active and passive abduction limited to 90 degrees. Palpation without point tenderness. Arm drop test negative
Vascular:	Brachial and radial pulses 2/4 bilaterally
Neuro:	Patient unable to perform left shoulder strength testing because of apprehension
	Bilateral upper extremities sensory intact to sharp/dull and light touch
	Reflexes 2/4 brachial, radial and brachioradialis bilaterally

Assessment

1) Adhesive capsulitis
2) Somatic dysfunction
3) Rule out arthritis
4) Doubt rotator cuff injury
5) Doubt ACS but with risk factors
6) Diabetes

Plan

1) Ibuprofen 600 mg three times a day with food × 5 days
2) OMM—Spencer technique performed
3) Left shoulder X-ray, EKG, CBC, Bun/creat, Hgb A1c
4) Instructed on ROM exercises. Offered work excuse; patient declined
5) Return to office in 5 days for follow-up and results   Jennifer Lin OMS-IV

Case 3

Patient Name: Ida Kno
Clinical Setting: Primary Care Outpatient Office Visit
CC: A 76 y/o female is brought into your office by her daughter for forgetfulness.

Vital Signs
Blood pressure: 158/88
Respirations: 12 per minute
Temperature: 98.8°F
Pulse: 72 bpm
Weight: 112 lbs
Height: 5' 4"

NOTES:

Subjective

Objective

Assessment

Plan

CC: A 76 y/o female is brought into your office by her daughter for forgetfulness.
Daughter answered the majority of the questions (mother's answers are in bold type)

		History		✓
	1	Introduces self and explains role of provider.		✓
	2	Properly washes hands before touching the patient (15-sec wash and turns off with towel).		✓
	3	Opening question: What brings you in today?	**My daughter**. (Daughter answers, "Mom's getting forgetful.")	✓
Chronology/ Onset	4	When did this **start**?	At least a year or more ago.	✓
	5	How has it **changed**?	It's getting worse.	✓
Description	6	**Describe** or give an **example** of the forgetfulness.	She can never find things.	✓
Intensity	7	How has it affected her **activities of daily living**?	I have to take her everywhere.	✓
Exacerbations	8	Does anything make this **worse**?	Not that I've noticed.	✓
Remissions	9	Does anything make this **better**?	She seems better in the mornings.	✓
Symptoms associated	10	**Slurred speech, facial droop**?	She can't find the right words.	✓
	11	**Numbness/tingling/weakness**?	No.	✓
	12	**Fever or chills**?	No.	✓
	13	Has she **fallen** or **hurt** herself?	No.	
	14	**Anxiety**?	Yes, she's so restless.	
	15	**Depression**?	She seems down all the time.	
	16	**Sleeping**?	She's up a lot throughout the night.	✓
	17	**Appetite**?	We have to remind her to eat.	
Social Hx	18	Do you **smoke**?	**No.**	✓
	19	Do you drink **alcohol**?	**No.**	✓
	20	**Caffeine**?	**I like tea.**	✓
	21	What is her **occupation**?	She stayed at home and raised us.	
Medical Hx	22	Does she have any medical conditions?	She has arthritis.	✓
Allergies	23	Does she have any allergies?	No.	✓
Surgical Hx	24	Has she had any surgeries?	No.	✓
Hosp Hx	25	Has she ever been hospitalized?	No.	✓
Family Hx	26	Medical conditions that run in the family?	Her mother didn't know us in the end.	✓
Medications	27	Is she on any medications?	She takes arthritis medicine.	✓
	28	Do you know the name?	No, I don't.	✓

Physical Examination ✓

	29	Informs patient that the physical exam is to begin and asks permission.		✓
	30	Rewashes hand before touching patient if candidate has recontaminated them.		✓
Vitals	31	Repeats BP with correct technique.	**BP 150/68**	✗
	32	Appropriate size cuff		
	33	Applied correctly placing cuff on bare arm		
General	34	General assessment	**Alert, no apparent distress, thin**	
Neurologic	35	Cranial nerves	**CN II–XII intact**	
	36	Muscle strength: B/l upper and lower extremities	**5/5 throughout**	
	37	Sensation: Sharp/dull b/l upper/lower extremities	**Intact throughout**	
	38	Reflexes: bilateral upper and lower extremities	**3/4 R arm/leg and 2/4 L arm/leg**	
	39	Babinski's	**Up going right, down going left**	
	40	Cerebellar function: Romberg, Finger/nose, RAM	**Intact**	
Neck	41	Auscultation for bruits	**Left carotid bruit**	✓
	42	Palpation of thyroid	**No thyromegaly**	✓
Respiratory	43	Auscultation performed on bare skin	**Clear to auscultation**	✓
	44	Through complete inspiration and expiration		
	45	Symmetrically		
	46	At least 2 anterior levels, 1 lateral, and 3 posterior		
Cardiac	47	Auscultation performed on bare skin	**RR without murmurs, rubs, gallops**	✓
	48	Areas: aortic, pulmonic, tricuspid, and mitral		
Mental Status	49	Assesses orientation.	**Oriented to person only**	
Assessment	50	Presents patient/family with a proposed diagnosis.	**Dementia**	
Plan	51	MTHR: Testing (CT scan, carotid ultrasound, labs), holistic (agency resources), MMSE		
(MOTHRR)	52	Return plan: Devises and explains a follow-up plan with the patient and family.		
	53	Thanks the patient and asks if there are any questions.		✓

Humanistic Evaluation Y/N

	Y/N
Did the candidate present in a self-caring manner (e.g., hair control, clothing, cleanliness, aroma, etc.)?	
Did the candidate make periodic eye contact?	
Was the candidate's language clear and EASY to understand?	
Did the candidate have any substance in his or her mouth during the session?	
Did the candidate exhibit body language that would make you feel the candidate was communicating with you?	
Was the candidate enthusiastic?	
Did the candidate exhibit pride in his or her efforts?	
Did the candidate make any comment regarding your lifestyle (e.g., your work, family, activities, etc.)?	
Did the candidate express any humanistic statement recognizing your concerns?	
Did the candidate explain the medical problem and offer you a possible diagnosis?	
Did the candidate suggest a treatment plan that you could understand?	
Did the candidate inquire whether you might want to consult with family members or others about your visit?	
Did the candidate present as if he or she were a competent interviewer?	
Did the candidate ask you if you had any questions?	
Did the candidate thank you?	

Case 4

Patient Name: Ness Tinter
Clinical Setting: Primary Care Outpatient Office Visit
CC: A 26 y/o female presents c/o foot pain.

Vital Signs
Blood pressure: 112/58
Respirations: 12 per minute
Temperature: 98.8°F
Pulse: 72 bpm
Weight: 124 lbs
Height: 5' 4"

NOTES:

Subjective

Objective

Assessment

Plan

CC: A 26 y/o female presents c/o foot pain.

History			✓	
	1	Introduces self and explains role of provider.		✓
	2	Properly washes hands before touching the patient (15-sec wash and turns off with towel).		✓
	3	Opening question: What brings you in today?	I hurt my ankle.	✓
Onset	4	**When** did it happen?	Yesterday.	✓
	5	**How/what** were you **doing** at the time?	I stepped off a curb and twisted it.	✓
Chronology	6	Has this ever happened **before**?	Yes. This is probably the third time.	
	7	**When**?	I twisted it the first time 6 years ago.	
	8	**How was it treated**?	My doctor tells me to take ibuprofen. They usually wrap it. I've also been to physical therapy twice.	
Description/ Duration	9	**Where** is the pain?	The outside of my right ankle.	✓
	10	**Describe** the pain.	It's sharp.	✓
Intensity	11	How severe is it, on a scale from **1 to 10**?	About a 5.	✓
Exacerbation	12	What makes it **worse**?	Trying to walk on it.	✓
Remission	13	What makes it **better**?	Ibuprofen helps.	✓
	14	**How much** did you take?	600 mg.	✓
	15	How **often** are you taking it?	Every 3 hours.	✓
Symptoms associated	16	Any **bruising**?	Yes.	✓
	17	Any **swelling**?	It was swollen last night.	✓
	18	**Numbness or tingling**?	Maybe a little along the side.	✓
Social Hx	19	Do you **smoke or use tobacco**?	Yes.	✓
(FED TACOS)	20	**How much** a day?	About 5 cigarettes a day.	✓
	21	For **how long**?	About 5 years.	✓
	22	Do you drink **alcohol**?	No.	✓
	23	What is your **occupation**?	I'm in grad school and waitress at night.	✓
	24	**FDLMP**?	About a week ago.	
Medical Hx	25	Do you have any medical conditions?	I have reflux.	✓
Allergies	26	Do you have any allergies?	No.	✓
Surgical Hx	27	Have you had any surgeries?	No.	✓
Hosp Hx	28	Have you ever been hospitalized?	No.	✓
Family Hx	29	Medical conditions that run in the family?	High cholesterol.	✓
Medications	30	Are you on any medications?	Zantac.	✓
	31	How much?	Once a day	✓
	32	How many milligrams?	I'm not sure.	✓

Physical Examination ✓

	33	Informs patient that the physical exam is to begin and asks permission.	✓
	34	Rewashes hand before touching patient if candidate has recontaminated them.	✓
MS	35	Covers patient with a sheet from waist down.	
	36	Raises sheet to expose bilateral lower extremities.	
	37	Inspection of right ankle	**Ecchymosis inferior lateral malleolus**	✓
	38	Comparison to left ankle	
	39	Active range of motion right ankle	**Limited inversion**	✓
	40	Passive range of motion	**Limited inversion due to pain.**	✓
	41	Palpation	**Tenderness R lat ligament complex**	✓
Neurologic	42	Sensory exam light touch or sharp vs. dull	**Intact**	
Vascular	43	Peripheral pulses	**Intact**	
Position change	44	Helps patient with position change to standing.	✓
	45	Assess gait.	**Patient walks with limp on right.**	✓
Assessment	46	Presents patient with a proposed diagnosis.	**Achilles injury, sprain, or rupture**	✓
Plan	47	MTHR: Pain control (reduce ibuprofen), testing, holistic (RICE), referral	✓
(MOTHRR)	48	Explains and offers OMM.	✓
	49	Performs OMM appropriately (no HVLA).	✓
	50	Return plan: Devises and explains a follow-up plan with the patient.	✓
	51	Thanks the patient and asks the patient if she has any questions.	✓

Humanistic Evaluation — Y/N

	Y/N
Did the candidate present in a self-caring manner (e.g., hair control, clothing, cleanliness, aroma, etc.)?	
Did the candidate make periodic eye contact?	
Was the candidate's language clear and EASY to understand?	
Did the candidate have any substance in his or her mouth during the session?	
Did the candidate exhibit body language that would make you feel the candidate was communicating with you?	
Was the candidate enthusiastic?	
Did the candidate exhibit pride in his or her efforts?	
Did the candidate make any comment regarding your lifestyle (e.g., your work, family, activities, etc.)?	
Did the candidate express any humanistic statement recognizing your concerns?	
Did the candidate explain the medical problem and offer you a possible diagnosis?	
Did the candidate suggest a treatment plan that you could understand?	
Did the candidate inquire whether you might want to consult with family members or others about your visit?	
Did the candidate present as if he or she were a competent interviewer?	
Did the candidate ask you if you had any questions?	
Did the candidate thank you?	

Case 5

Patient Name:	Chester Paine
Clinical Setting:	Emergency Room
CC:	A 62 y/o Caucasian male presents with chest pain.

Vital Signs

Blood pressure:	180/104
Respirations:	20 per minute
Temperature:	97.9°F
Pulse:	88 bpm
Weight:	230 lbs
Height:	6' 1"

NOTES:

Subjective

Objective

Assessment

Plan

CC: A 62 y/o Caucasian male presents with chest pain.

History			✓
	1 Introduces self and explains role of provider.		✓
	2 Properly washes hands before touching the patient (15-sec wash and turns off with towel).		✓
	3 Opening question: What brings you in today?	I was having chest pain.	✓
Chronology/ Onset	4 When did it **start**?	An hour ago.	✓
	5 Was the onset **sudden** or **gradual**?	Sudden.	
	6 What were you **doing when it started**?	Walking around the block.	✓
Duration	7 How **long** did the pain **last**?	Twenty minutes.	✓
	8 Did you ever have this **before**?	Yes.	✓
	9 When?	All last year . . . whenever I walk my dog.	✓
	10 How long does the pain **usually last**?	Three to 4 minutes.	✓
	11 Has it **changed in any way**?	I can't even walk a block anymore.	
Description	12 **Describe** the pain.	Sharp, aching, deep.	✓
	13 **Where** is the pain?	*Points just above the xiphoid process*	✓
	14 Does it **radiate/go** anywhere?	No.	✓
Intensity	15 How severe is it, on a scale from **1 to 10**?	It was a 7 or 8.	✓
Exacerbation	16 What makes it **worse**?	Well, anytime I overexert myself really.	
	17 Have you ever had this pain **at rest**?	Just in the past month or so.	
Remission	18 What makes it **better**?	Resting for a few minutes usually works.	
Symptoms associated	19 **Sweating**?	Sometimes, but just on my face.	✓
	20 **Nausea or vomiting**?	No.	✓
	21 **Shortness of breath**?	Only a little. Just when I get the pain.	✓
	22 **Dyspepsia**?	No.	
	23 **Cough**?	No.	
Social Hx	24 What does your **diet** look like?	I eat whatever I want.	
(FED TACOS)	25 Do you **exercise**?	Just walking the dog.	
	26 Do you **smoke**?	Yes.	✓
	27 **How much** do you smoke a day?	Two packs a day.	✓
	28 **How long** have you been smoking?	Twenty-five years.	✓
	29 Do you drink **alcohol**?	Yes.	✓
	30 How many drinks a day?	Two to 3 beers a day.	✓
	31 Do you use any **drugs**?	Ah, come on, Doc.	
	32 What is your **occupation**?	I'm an architect.	✓
Medical Hx	33 Do you have any medical conditions?	My blood pressure and cholesterol are high.	✓
Allergies	34 Do you have any allergies?	No.	✓
Surg Hx	35 Have you had any surgeries?	No.	✓
Hosp Hx	36 Have you ever been hospitalized?	No.	✓
Family Hx	37 Medical conditions that run in the family?	My parents had heart attacks in their 50s.	✓
Medications	38 Are you on any medications?	Hydrochlorothiazide and lovastatin.	✓
	39 Do you know the doses?	No.	✓
	40 How many times a day do you take each?	I just take one of each once a day.	

Physical Examination ✓

	41	Informs patient that the physical exam is to begin and asks permission.	
	42	Rewashes hand before touching patient if candidate has recontaminated them.	
Vitals	43	Repeats BP with correct technique.	BP 176/96	✓
	44	Appropriate size cuff		✓
	45	Applied correctly placing cuff on bare arm		✓
General	46	Assess for **distress**.	**No apparent distress**
Neck	47	Assess for **JVD**.	**No JVD**
	48	Auscultation for carotid bruit.	**No bruit**
Cardiac	49	Inspection: properly exposes the chest	**No heave or visible PMI**
	50	Auscultation performed on bare skin	**Reg rhythm w/o murmur, rub, or gallop**
	51	Areas: aortic, pulmonic, tricuspid, and mitral	
	52	Palpation for PMI	**Anterior axillary line 5th ICS**
Respiratory	53	Auscultation performed on bare skin	**Clear to auscultation**	✓
	54	Through complete inspiration and expiration	
	55	Symmetrically	
	56	At least 2 anterior levels, 1 lateral, and 3 posterior	
Abdominal	57	Helps patient with position changes.	
	58	Covers lower extremities with a sheet during the exam.	
	59	Inspection: properly exposes the abdomen	**No masses**
	60	Auscultation prior to palpation	**NABS without bruit**
	61	Palpation of size of abdominal aorta	**No pulsitile masses**
Assessment	62	Presents patient with a proposed diagnosis.	**Angina**	✓
Plan	63	MTHR: Aspirin, beta blocker, X-ray, ECG, labs, referral		✓
(MOTHRR)	64	Advises admission and cardiac evaluation.		✓
	65	Thanks the patient and asks if there are any questions.		✓

Humanistic Evaluation Y/N

	Y/N
Did the candidate present in a self-caring manner (e.g., hair control, clothing, cleanliness, aroma, etc.)?	
Did the candidate make periodic eye contact?	
Was the candidate's language clear and EASY to understand?	
Did the candidate have any substance in his or her mouth during the session?	
Did the candidate exhibit body language that would make you feel the candidate was communicating with you?	
Was the candidate enthusiastic?	
Did the candidate exhibit pride in his or her efforts?	
Did the candidate make any comment regarding your lifestyle (e.g., your work, family, activities, etc.)?	
Did the candidate express any humanistic statement recognizing your concerns?	
Did the candidate explain the medical problem and offer you a possible diagnosis?	
Did the candidate suggest a treatment plan that you could understand?	
Did the candidate inquire whether you might want to consult with family members or others about your visit?	
Did the candidate present as if he or she were a competent interviewer?	
Did the candidate ask you if you had any questions?	
Did the candidate thank you?	

Case 6

Patient Name:	Jim Zahurtin
Clinical Setting:	Emergency Room
CC:	A 35 y/o Caucasian male presents with abdominal pain.

Vital Signs

Blood pressure:	118/64
Respirations:	24 per minute
Temperature:	102°F
Pulse:	104 bpm
Weight:	202 lbs
Height:	5'9"

NOTES:

Subjective

Objective

Assessment

Plan

CC: A 35 y/o Caucasian male presents with abdominal pain.

History			✓
	1 Introduces self and explains role of provider.		✓
	2 Properly washes hands before touching the patient (15-sec wash and turns off with towel).		✓
	3 Opening question: What brings you in today?	My stomach hurts.	✓
Chronology Onset	4 **When** did it **start**?	Last night.	✓
	5 Have you had this **before**?	No.	✓
	6 What were you **doing**?	Getting ready for bed.	✓
	7 Have there been any **changes** in the pain?	It feels like it's moving farther down.	
Description	8 **Where** is it?	*Points to RLQ*	✓
Duration	9 Does it **radiate (go)** anywhere?	Sort of into my back.	
	10 **Where** to?	*Points to right lumbar region*	
	11 **Describe** the pain.	It's sharp and stabbing.	✓
	12 **Constant** or **come and go**?	Constant.	✓
Intensity	13 How severe is it, on a scale from **1 to 10**?	A 9.	✓
Exacerbation	14 What makes it **worse**?	Pushing on my stomach.	✓
Remission	15 Did you try anything to make it **better**?	I tried Tums, but they didn't help.	✓
Symptoms associated	16 **Nausea or vomiting**?	Once this morning.	✓
	17 Have you been **eating well**?	I don't feel like eating.	
	18 **Diarrhea or constipation**?	A little diarrhea this morning.	✓
	19 Was there any **blood** or **mucus** in it?	No.	✓
	20 **Fever** or **chills**?	I do feel a little warm.	✓
	21 **Burning with urination**?	No.	✓
	22 **Blood** in the urine?	No.	
Social Hx	23 Do you **smoke**?	No.	✓
	24 Do you **drink**?	Yes.	✓
	25 **How much** a day?	Two beers, once or twice a month.	✓
	26 Do you use any **drugs**?	No.	✓
Medical Hx	27 Do you have any medical conditions?	I have hypothyroidism.	✓
Allergies	28 Do you have any allergies?	No.	✓
Surg Hx	29 Have you had any surgeries?	No.	✓
Hosp Hx	30 Have you ever been hospitalized?	No.	✓
Family Hx	31 Medical conditions that run in the family?	Some high blood pressure.	✓
	32 Family members/contacts with same symptoms?	No.	
Medications	33 Are you on any medications?	Synthroid.	✓
	34 How many milligrams a day?	0.15, I think.	✓

Physical Examination ✓

	35	Informs patient that the physical exam is to begin and asks permission.		
	36	Rewashes hand before touching patient if candidate has recontaminated them.		
General	37	Assess for **distress**.		
	38	**Position of comfort**		
HEENT	39	Inspect for icterus	**No icterus**	
Respiratory	40	Auscultation performed on bare skin	**Clear to auscultation**	✓
	41	Through complete inspiration and expiration		
	42	Symmetrically		
	43	At least 2 anterior levels, 1 lateral, and 3 posterior		
Cardiac	44	Auscultation performed on bare skin	**RR without murmurs, rubs, gallops**	✓
	45	Areas: aortic, pulmonic, tricuspid, and mitral		
Abdominal	46	Helps patient to supine position.		
	47	Drapes lower extremities with sheet.		
	48	Inspection: properly exposes the abdomen	**Rounded**	✓
	49	Auscultation prior to palpation	**Hypoactive bowel sounds**	✓
	50	Percussion: four quadrants	**Diffuse tenderness prevents exam**	✓
	51	Palpation watching facial expression	**Tenderness greatest in the RLQ**	✓
	52	Rebound, rigidity, guarding	**Positive**	
	53	Rovsing's sign: pain in RLQ with palpation of LLQ	**Positive**	
Rectal	54	Advises patient that rectal exam is recommended.	**Not performed on SP**	
Assessment	55	Presents patient with a proposed diagnosis.	**Appendicitis**	
Plan	56	MTHR: Antibiotics, imaging, pain control after surgical consult		
(MOTHRR)	57	Advises admission and surgical evaluation.		
	58	Thanks the patient and asks if there are any questions.		

Humanistic Evaluation Y/N

Did the candidate present in a self-caring manner (e.g., hair control, clothing, cleanliness, aroma, etc.)?	
Did the candidate make periodic eye contact?	
Was the candidate's language clear and EASY to understand?	
Did the candidate have any substance in his or her mouth during the session?	
Did the candidate exhibit body language that would make you feel the candidate was communicating with you?	
Was the candidate enthusiastic?	
Did the candidate exhibit pride in his or her efforts?	
Did the candidate make any comment regarding your lifestyle (e.g., your work, family, activities, etc.)?	
Did the candidate express any humanistic statement recognizing your concerns?	
Did the candidate explain the medical problem and offer you a possible diagnosis?	
Did the candidate suggest a treatment plan that you could understand?	
Did the candidate inquire whether you might want to consult with family members or others about your visit?	
Did the candidate present as if he or she were a competent interviewer?	
Did the candidate ask you if you had any questions?	
Did the candidate thank you?	

Case 7

Patient Name:	Torrie Esper
Clinical Setting:	Family Practice Office
CC:	A 35 y/o Caucasian male presents with shortness of breath.

Vital Signs

Blood pressure:	122/68
Respirations:	16 per minute
Temperature:	98.6°F
Pulse:	72 bpm
Weight:	180 lbs
Height:	6' 3"

NOTES:

Subjective

Objective

Assessment

Plan

CC: A 35 y/o Caucasian male presents with shortness of breath.

History			✓
	1	Introduces self and explains role of provider.	✓
	2	Properly washes hands before touching the patient (15-sec wash and off with towel).	✓
	3	Opening question: What brings you in today?	I get short of breath now and then.	✓
Chronology/ Onset	4	Are you short of breath **right now**?	No.	
	5	**When** did this start?	Over the last couple of years, I guess.	✓
	6	Are you **doing anything** when it happens?	It happens when I go outside and it's cold.	✓
	7	Does it come on **suddenly or gradually**?	More gradually.	
	8	Did you ever have this **before**?	I had something similar when I was a kid.	
	9	How was it **treated**?	I took some sort of aerosol medicine.	
Description	10	Could you **describe your shortness of breath**?	It feels like I can't let my breath out.	
Duration	11	**How long does it last** when it happens?	An hour or so, if I get out of the cold.	
Intensity	12	How does this affect your **daily activities**?	I just don't go outside that much.	✓
Exacerbation	13	Does anything make it **worse**?	Dusty houses cause the same thing.	✓
Remission	14	What makes it **better**?	Just keeping out of the cold.	✓
Symptoms associated	15	**Wheezing**?	Yes, I wheeze every time it happens.	✓
	16	**Cough**?	Just when it happens.	✓
	17	**Sputum production**?	No.	✓
	18	**Chest pain**?	No.	✓
	19	**Fever or chills**?	No.	✓
Social Hx	20	What does your **diet** look like?	I eat on the run.	
(FED TACOS)	21	Do you **exercise**?	I lift weights three days a week.	
	22	Do you **smoke**?	A little.	✓
	23	**How much** a day?	About a half pack.	✓
	24	**How many years**?	About 15 years or so.	
	25	Do you drink **alcohol**?	No.	✓
	26	Do you drink **caffeine**?	I have couple cups of coffee a day.	✓
	27	What is your **occupation**?	I'm a mortgage broker.	✓
Medical Hx	28	Do you have any medical conditions?	No.	✓
Allergies	29	Do you have any allergies?	A little seasonal runny nose.	✓
Surg Hx	30	Have you had any surgeries?	No.	✓
Hosp Hx	31	Have you ever been hospitalized?	No.	✓
Family Hx	32	Medical conditions that run in the family?	There were some breathing problems.	✓
	33	Do you know what those problems were?	Asthma, I think.	✓
Medications	34	Are you on any medications?	Benadryl.	✓
	35	How many pills a day?	One or two.	✓
	36	How many milligrams?	25 or 50 mg. I'm not sure.	

Physical Examination ✓

				✓
	37	Informs patient that the physical exam is to begin and asks permission.		
	38	Rewashes hand before touching patient if candidate has recontaminated them.		
Gen Assessment	39	Inspection	**Tall, thin; in no apparent distress**	
Skin	40	Inspection of skin and nails	**No cyanosis, pallor, or clubbing**	✓
HEENT	41	Inspection: otoscopic exam	**Nasal mucosa pallor without polyps**	
Respiratory	42	Auscultation performed on bare skin	**Clear to auscultation**	✓
	43	Through complete inspiration and expiration		✓
	44	Symmetrically		✓
	45	At least 2 anterior levels, 1 lateral, and 3 posterior		✓
Cardiac	46	Auscultation performed on bare skin	**RR without murmurs, rubs, gallops**	✓
	47	Areas: aortic, pulmonic, tricuspid, and mitral		
Assessment	48	Presents patient with a proposed diagnosis.	**Asthma, COPD**	
Plan	49	MTHR: peak flow meter, imaging, smoking cessation		
(MOTHRR)	50	Explains and offers OMM.		✓
	51	Performs OMM appropriately (no HVLA).		✓
	52	Return plan: Devises and explains a follow-up plan with the patient.		
	53	Thanks the patient and asks if there are any questions.		

Humanistic Evaluation Y/N

	Y/N
Did the candidate present in a self-caring manner (e.g., hair control, clothing, cleanliness, aroma, etc.)?	
Did the candidate make periodic eye contact?	
Was the candidate's language clear and EASY to understand?	
Did the candidate have any substance in his or her mouth during the session?	
Did the candidate exhibit body language that would make you feel the candidate was communicating with you?	
Was the candidate enthusiastic?	
Did the candidate exhibit pride in his or her efforts?	
Did the candidate make any comment regarding your lifestyle (e.g., your work, family, activities, etc.)?	
Did the candidate express any humanistic statement recognizing your concerns?	
Did the candidate explain the medical problem and offer you a possible diagnosis?	
Did the candidate suggest a treatment plan that you could understand?	
Did the candidate inquire whether you might want to consult with family members or others about your visit?	
Did the candidate present as if he or she were a competent interviewer?	
Did the candidate ask you if you had any questions?	
Did the candidate thank you?	

Case 8

Patient Name:	Sakrel Torres
Clinical Setting:	Primary Care Office
CC:	An 88 y/o male presents with back pain.

Vital Signs

Blood pressure:	152/72
Respirations:	16 per minute
Temperature:	98.2°F
Pulse:	70 bpm
Weight:	166 lbs
Height:	5'9"

NOTES:

Subjective

Objective

Assessment

Plan

CC: An 88 y/o male presents with back pain.

History			✓
	1 Introduces self and explains role of provider.		✓
	2 Properly washes hands before touching the patient (15-sec wash and turns off with towel).		✓
	3 Opening question: What brings you in today?	My back hurts.	✓
Chronology/ Onset	4 **How** did you hurt it?	I slipped on the rug and fell on my butt.	✓
	5 **When** did that happen?	Last night.	✓
	6 Did this ever happen **before**?	No.	✓
Description/ Duration	7 **Describe** the pain.	I don't know, it just hurts.	✓
	8 **Where** is the pain?	Right in the middle, on my butt bone.	✓
Intensity	9 Rate the **intensity** on a scale of 1 to 10?	A 4 or 5.	✓
Exacerbation	10 What makes it **worse**?	Sitting on it.	✓
Remission	11 What makes it **better**?	Nothing, that's why I'm here.	✓
Symptoms associated	12 Any **swelling**?	I can't see back there.	
	13 Any change to your **bowel or bladder** habits?	No. I'm as regular as Old Faithful.	✓
	14 Any **incontinence**?	No.	
	15 Any **numbness, weakness, or tingling**?	No.	✓
Social Hx	16 Do you **exercise**?	Don't have to. I'm too busy.	
	17 Do you **smoke**?	No.	✓
	18 Do you drink **alcohol**?	No.	✓
	19 What is your **occupation**?	I'm a farmer.	✓
Medical Hx	20 Do you have any medical conditions?	I got high blood pressure and gout.	✓
Allergies	21 Do you have any allergies?	No.	✓
Surg Hx	22 Have you had any surgeries?	No.	✓
Hosp Hx	23 Have you ever been hospitalized?	No.	✓
Family Hx	24 Medical conditions that run in the family?	I can't remember anything in particular.	✓
Medications	25 Are you on any medications?	A water pill and something for the gout.	✓
	26 Do you know the names or doses?	No. I just take what I'm told.	✓

Physical Examination ✓

			✓
	27	Informs patient that the physical exam is to begin and asks permission.	
	28	Rewashes hand before touching patient if candidate has recontaminated them.	
Vitals	29	Repeats BP with correct technique. **Repeat BP 138/84**	
	30	Appropriate size cuff	
	31	Applied correctly placing cuff on bare arm	
General	32	Assesses for distress, position of comfort. **Patient standing, will not sit**	
Cardiac	33	Auscultation performed on bare skin **Regular rhythm w/o murmur, rub, gallop**	✓
	34	Areas: aortic, pulmonic, tricuspid, and mitral	
Respiratory	35	Auscultation performed on bare skin **Clear to auscultation**	
	36	Through complete inspiration and expiration	
	37	Symmetrically	
	38	At least 2 anterior levels, 1 lateral, and 3 posterior	
MS	39	Inspection of area of trauma **Ecchymosis at inferior sacrum**	✓
	40	Palpation **Tenderness at midsacrum**	✓
	41	Osteopathic examination **Right on right sacral torsion**	✓
Neuro	42	Lower extremity reflexes **2/4 bilateral patellar and Achilles**	
	43	Lower extremity strength **5/5 hip and knee flexion and extension**	
Rectal	44	Advises SP that rectal exam is recommended. **Exam NOT performed on SP**	✓
Assessment	45	Presents patient with a proposed diagnosis. **Sacral torsion and contusion**	
Plan	46	MTHR: Pain control, holistic (RICE), imaging, BP follow-up	
(MOTHRR)	47	Performs appropriate manipulation.	✓
	48	Explains and offers OMM.	✓
	49	Performs OMM appropriately (no HVLA).	✓
	50	Return plan: Devises and explains a follow-up plan with the patient.	
	51	Thanks the patient and asks if there are any questions.	

Humanistic Evaluation Y/N

	Y/N
Did the candidate present in a self-caring manner (e.g., hair control, clothing, cleanliness, aroma, etc.)?	
Did the candidate make periodic eye contact?	
Was the candidate's language clear and EASY to understand?	
Did the candidate have any substance in his or her mouth during the session?	
Did the candidate exhibit body language that would make you feel the candidate was communicating with you?	
Was the candidate enthusiastic?	
Did the candidate exhibit pride in his or her efforts?	
Did the candidate make any comment regarding your lifestyle (e.g., your work, family, activities, etc.)?	
Did the candidate express any humanistic statement recognizing your concerns?	
Did the candidate explain the medical problem and offer you a possible diagnosis?	
Did the candidate suggest a treatment plan that you could understand?	
Did the candidate inquire whether you might want to consult with family members or others about your visit?	
Did the candidate present as if he or she were a competent interviewer?	
Did the candidate ask you if you had any questions?	
Did the candidate thank you?	

Case 9

Patient Name:	Ester Wilhapen
Clinical Setting:	Family Practice Office
CC:	A 15 y/o female presents for "a burn on my forehead."

Vital Signs

Blood pressure:	108/70
Respirations:	14 per minute
Temperature:	98°F
Pulse:	76 bpm
Weight:	180 lbs
Height:	5'6"

NOTES:

Subjective

Objective

Assessment

Plan

CC: A 15 y/o female presents for "a burn on my forehead."

History			✓
	1 Introduces self and explains role of provider.		✓
	2 Properly washes hands before touching the patient (15-sec wash and turns off with towel).		✓
	3 Opening question: What brings you in today?	I burnt my forehead.	✓
Chronology/ Onset	4 **When** did this happen?	Earlier today.	✓
	5 Did you ever have this **before**?	No.	✓
	6 What were you **doing** when it happened?	Curling my hair.	✓
Exacerbation	7 Does anything make it **worse**?	Touching it.	✓
Remission	8 What makes it **better**?	My grandma said to put butter on it.	✓
Symptoms associated	9 **Bleeding**?	No.	✓
	10 **Discharge**?	A little clear drainage.	✓
	11 **Pain**?	Yes.	✓
Intensity	12 How severe is it, on a scale from **1 to 10**?	About a 6.	✓
Social Hx	13 What does your **diet** look like?	I'm 15. I eat a lot of fast food.	
(FED TACOS)	14 Do you **exercise**?	Not really.	
	15 Do you **smoke**?	A little.	✓
	16 **How much** is a little?	A couple on weekends.	✓
	17 **How long** have you been smoking?	Only a year or so.	✓
	18 Do you drink **alcohol**?	No.	✓
	19 Do you use any **drugs**?	No.	✓
Medical Hx	20 Do you have any medical conditions?	Diabetes.	✓
Allergies	21 Do you have any allergies?	No.	✓
Surg Hx	22 Have you had any surgeries?	No.	✓
Hosp Hx	23 Have you ever been hospitalized?	No.	✓
Family Hx	24 Medical conditions that run in the family?	Diabetes.	✓
Medications	25 Are you on any medications?	Just insulin.	✓
	26 Do you know the doses?	I'm on a pump.	✓
	27 How many times a day do you take each?	It's automatic.	✓

Physical Examination ✓

			✓
	28	Informs patient that the physical exam is to begin and asks permission.	✓
	29	Rewashes hand before touching patient if candidate has recontaminated them.	✓
Skin	30	Inspection	**3' × 1" denuded epidermis R forehead with surrounding erythema and clear serous drainage** ✓
	31	Palpation	**Nontender around borders** ✓
Cardiac	32	Auscultation performed on bare skin	**Reg rhythm w/o murmur, rub, gallop** ✓
	33	Areas: aortic, pulmonic, tricuspid, and mitral	
Respiratory	34	Auscultation performed on bare skin	**Clear to auscultation** ✓
	35	Through complete inspiration and expiration	✓
	36	Symmetrically	✓
	37	At least 2 anterior levels, 1 lateral, and 3 posterior	✓
Assessment	38	Presents patient with a proposed diagnosis.	**First-degree burn** ✓
Plan	39	MTHR: Topical antibiotic, pain control, holistic (smoking cessation, diet, exercise), educates on wound care	✓
(MOTHRR)	40	Return plan: Devises and explains a follow-up plan with the patient.	
	41	Thanks the patient and asks if there are any questions.	

Humanistic Evaluation Y/N

	Y/N
Did the candidate present in a self-caring manner (e.g., hair control, clothing, cleanliness, aroma, etc.)?	
Did the candidate make periodic eye contact?	
Was the candidate's language clear and EASY to understand?	
Did the candidate have any substance in his or her mouth during the session?	
Did the candidate exhibit body language that would make you feel the candidate was communicating with you?	
Was the candidate enthusiastic?	
Did the candidate exhibit pride in his or her efforts?	
Did the candidate make any comment regarding your lifestyle (e.g., your work, family, activities, etc.)?	
Did the candidate express any humanistic statement recognizing your concerns?	
Did the candidate explain the medical problem and offer you a possible diagnosis?	
Did the candidate suggest a treatment plan that you could understand?	
Did the candidate inquire whether you might want to consult with family members or others about your visit?	
Did the candidate present as if he or she were a competent interviewer?	
Did the candidate ask you if you had any questions?	
Did the candidate thank you?	

Case 10

Patient Name: Farah Grates
Clinical Setting: Family Practice Office
CC: A 21 y/o female complaining of a cold.

Vital Signs
Blood pressure: 110/60
Respirations: 16 per minute
Temperature: 100.1°F
Pulse: 88 bpm
Weight: 128 lbs
Height: 5'9"

NOTES:

Subjective

Objective

Assessment

Plan

CC: A 21 y/o female complaining of a cold.

History			✓
	1	Introduces self and explains role of provider.	✓
	2	Properly washes hands before touching the patient (15-sec wash and turns off with towel).	✓
	3	Opening question: What brings you in today?	I've got a cold.	✓
Chronology/ Onset	4	When did it **start**?	About 3 days ago.	✓
	5	Was the onset **sudden** or **gradual**?	I guess gradual.	
	6	Did you ever have this **before**?	I had the same thing last year.	✓
	7	How was it treated?	I think they gave me an antibiotic.	
Description	8	**Describe** the "cold."	It's a runny nose and sore throat.	✓
Exacerbations	9	Anything make it **worse**?	It hurts more when I swallow.	✓
Remittance	10	Anything make it **better**?	Some cold tablets I took helped.	✓
	11	Do you know the **name** of them?	Tussi something.	✓
	12	**How much** did you take?	Two pills a couple of times yesterday.	
Symptoms associated	13	**Shortness of breath**?	No.	✓
	14	**Fever or chills**?	Both.	✓
	15	**Headache**?	Yes, right above my eyes.	✓
	16	**Sinus congestion/pressure**?	Yes.	
	17	**Ear pain**?	No, they just feel full.	.
	18	**Cough**?	No.	✓
	19	**Nausea or vomiting**?	No.	✓
Social Hx	20	Do you **smoke**?	No.	
(FED TACOS)	21	Do you drink **alcohol**?	No.	✓
	22	Do you use any **drugs**?	No.	✓
	23	What is your **occupation**?	I'm a senior in high school.	✓
Medical Hx	24	Do you have any medical conditions?	No, I'm pretty healthy.	✓
Allergies	25	Do you have any **allergies**?	I'm allergic to amoxicillin.	✓
	26	What happens when you take that?	I vomit.	✓
Surg Hx	27	Have you had any surgeries?	Do tubes in your ears count?	✓
Hosp Hx	28	Have you ever been hospitalized?	No.	✓
Family Hx	29	Medical conditions that run in the family?	My parents are pretty healthy.	✓
	30	Anyone you know with the same symptoms?	My little brother had this last week.	✓
Menstrual Hx	31	When was the **FDLMP**?	It started yesterday.	
Medications	32	Are you on any medications?	Just Benadryl when I need it.	✓

Physical Examination ✓

			✓
	33	Informs patient that the physical exam is to begin and asks permission.	
	34	Rewashes hands before touching patient if candidate has recontaminated them.	
General	35	Gen Alert, no respiratory distress	
Skin	36	Inspection	**No rash.**	
Sinuses	37	Inspection with transillumination	**Symmetrical.**	✓
	38	Palpation	**Mild maxillary sinus tenderness**	✓
Eyes	39	Inspection	**Conjunctive pink, sclera w/o injection**	✓
Ears	40	Otoscopic examination	**Tm's gray bilaterally, good light reflex**	✓
	41	Inverted otoscope with finger distended		✓
	42	Proper ear position—adult: up, back, out		✓
Nose	43	Inspection with light source	**Mucosal edema and clear exudate**	✓
Throat	44	Inspection with light source and tongue blade	**Pharyngeal erythema w/o exudate**	✓
Lymphatics	45	Palpation of cervical nodes	**Mild anterior cervical adenopathy**	✓
Respiratory	46	Auscultation performed on bare skin	**Clear to auscultation**	
	47	Through complete inspiration and expiration		
	48	Symmetrically		
	49	At least 2 anterior levels, 1 lateral, and 3 posterior		
Cardiac	50	Auscultation performed on bare skin	**RR without murmurs, rubs or gallops**	✓
	51	Areas: aortic, pulmonic, tricuspid, and mitral		
Assessment	52	Presents patient with a proposed diagnosis.	**URI**	
Plan	53	MTHR: Supportive therapy, throat culture, increase fluids, rest		
(MOTHRR)	54	Return plan: Devises and explains a follow-up plan with the patient.		
	55	Thanks the patient and asks if there are any questions.		

Humanistic Evaluation Y/N

	Y/N
Did the candidate present in a self-caring manner (e.g., hair control, clothing, cleanliness, aroma, etc.)?	
Did the candidate make periodic eye contact?	
Was the candidate's language clear and EASY to understand?	
Did the candidate have any substance in his or her mouth during the session?	
Did the candidate exhibit body language that would make you feel the candidate was communicating with you?	
Was the candidate enthusiastic?	
Did the candidate exhibit pride in his or her efforts?	
Did the candidate make any comment regarding your lifestyle (e.g., your work, family, activities, etc.)?	
Did the candidate express any humanistic statement recognizing your concerns?	
Did the candidate explain the medical problem and offer you a possible diagnosis?	
Did the candidate suggest a treatment plan that you could understand?	
Did the candidate inquire whether you might want to consult with family members or others about your visit?	
Did the candidate present as if he or she were a competent interviewer?	
Did the candidate ask you if you had any questions?	
Did the candidate thank you?	

Case 11

Patient Name: Eileen A. Little
Clinical Setting: Emergency Room
CC: An 82 y/o female is brought to the emergency room by ambulance.

Vital Signs
Blood pressure: 186/112
Respirations: 14 per minute
Temperature: 98.4°F
Pulse: 72 bpm
Weight: 136 lbs
Height: 5'7"

NOTES:

Subjective

Objective

Assessment

Plan

CC: An 82 y/o female is brought to the emergency room by ambulance.

History			✓
	1	Introduces self and explains role of provider.	✓
	2	Properly washes hands before touching the patient (15-sec wash and turns off with towel).	✓
	3	Opening question: What brings you in today? I feel weak.	✓
Chronology/ Onset	4	When did it **start**? While I was eating breakfast.	✓
	5	Was the onset **sudden** or **gradual**? It happened all of a sudden.	✓
	6	Did you ever have this **before**? No.	✓
Description	7	**Describe** the weakness. My whole right side went heavy.	✓
Intensity	8	**How Weak** are you? I couldn't pick up my coffee cup.	✓
Symptoms associated	9	**Slurred speech, facial droop**? No.	
	10	**Numbness/tingling**? My whole right side is numb, too.	✓
	11	**Visual changes**? I don't think so.	✓
	12	**Headache**? Not really.	✓
	13	**Palpitations or chest pain**? No.	
	14	**Shortness of breath**? No.	
	15	**Falls**? No.	✓
Social Hx	16	What does your **diet** look like? My daughter does my shopping.	
(FED TACOS)	17	Do you **exercise**? Well, I'm active.	
	18	Do you **smoke**? No.	✓
	19	Do you drink **alcohol**? No.	✓
	20	What is your **occupation**? I volunteer at the Veteran's Hospital.	✓
Medical Hx	21	Do you have any other **medical conditions**? I have high blood pressure.	✓
Allergies	22	Do you have any allergies? No.	✓
Surgical Hx	23	Have you had any surgeries? No.	✓
Hosp Hx	24	Have you ever been hospitalized? No.	✓
Family Hx	25	Medical conditions that run in the family? Not that I know of.	✓
Medications	26	Are you on any medications? I'm supposed to be.	✓
	27	Do you know the name? No, I don't.	✓
	28	Are you taking your medications? Not all the time.	✓

Physical Examination ✓

			✓
	29	Informs patient that the physical exam is to begin and asks permission.	
	30	Rewashes hand before touching patient if candidate has recontaminated them.	
Vitals	31	Repeats BP with correct technique. **BP 176/96**	
	32	Appropriate size cuff	
	33	Applied correctly placing cuff on bare arm.	
General	34	General assessment **Alert, no apparent distress**	
Neurologic	35	Assesses orientation. **Oriented × 3**	✓
	36	Cranial nerves **PERRLA, EOMI, no ptosis or facial droop, uvula midline, tongue midline**	✓
	37	Muscle strength **Weaker right arm and leg**	✓
	38	Sensation **Diminished right arm and leg**	✓
	39	Reflexes **Decreased reflexes R arm and leg**	✓
	40	Babinski **Up going right, down going left**	✓
Neck	41	Auscultation for bruits **Left carotid bruit**	✓
Cardiac	42	Auscultation performed on bare skin **Reg rhythm w/o murmur, rub, gallop**	✓
	43	Areas: aortic, pulmonic, tricuspid, and mitral	✓
Respiratory	44	Auscultation performed on bare skin **Clear to auscultation**	✓
	45	Through complete inspiration and expiration	✓
	46	Symmetrically	✓
	47	At least 2 anterior levels, 1 lateral, and 3 posterior	✓
Assessment	48	Presents patient with a proposed diagnosis. **CVA**	
Plan	49	MTHR: Stat imaging, labs, holistic (informs family), stroke team referral	
(MOTHRR)	50	Advises admission and stroke evaluation.	
	51	Thanks the patient and asks if there are any questions.	

Humanistic Evaluation Y/N

	Y/N
Did the candidate present in a self-caring manner (e.g., hair control, clothing, cleanliness, aroma, etc.)?	
Did the candidate make periodic eye contact?	
Was the candidate's language clear and EASY to understand?	
Did the candidate have any substance in his or her mouth during the session?	
Did the candidate exhibit body language that would make you feel the candidate was communicating with you?	
Was the candidate enthusiastic?	
Did the candidate exhibit pride in his or her efforts?	
Did the candidate make any comment regarding your lifestyle (e.g., your work, family, activities, etc.)?	
Did the candidate express any humanistic statement recognizing your concerns?	
Did the candidate explain the medical problem and offer you a possible diagnosis?	
Did the candidate suggest a treatment plan that you could understand?	
Did the candidate inquire whether you might want to consult with family members or others about your visit?	
Did the candidate present as if he or she were a competent interviewer?	
Did the candidate ask you if you had any questions?	
Did the candidate thank you?	

Case 12

Patient Name:	Polly Yoria
Clinical Setting:	Family Practice Office
CC:	A 24 y/o female presents for "UTI."

Vital Signs

Blood pressure:	116/76
Respirations:	14 per minute
Temperature:	98.4°F
Pulse:	76 bpm
Weight:	230 lbs
Height:	5'4"

NOTES:

Subjective

Objective

Assessment

Plan

CC: A 24 y/o female presents for "UTI."

History			✓
	1 Introduces self and explains role of provider.		✓
	2 Properly washes hands before touching the patient (15-sec wash and turns off with towel).		✓
	3 Opening question: What brings you in today?	I have a urinary tract infection.	✓
Chronology/ Onset	4 **When** did this start?	A couple of weeks ago.	✓
	5 Did you ever have this **before**?	Yes.	✓
	6 **How often** does it happen?	I had one about 2 years ago.	✓
Description	7 Could you **describe it**?	I have to pee all the time.	✓
Duration	8 **How often**?	About once every half an hour.	✓
	9 **How Many times to do get up at night**?	Four or five times a night.	✓
Exacerbation	10 Does anything make it **worse**?	Not really.	✓
Remission	11 What makes it **better**?	I tried cranberry juice, but it didn't work.	✓
Symptoms associated	12 **Burning with urination**?	No.	✓
	13 **Blood with urination**?	No.	
	14 **Vaginal discharge**?	No.	✓
	15 **Increased thirst**?	Yes, I am thirsty all the time.	
	16 **Increased hunger**?	More thirsty than hungry.	
	17 **Lightheadedness or dizziness**?	No.	
	18 **Weight loss or rain**	I've actually lost about 10 lbs.	
	19 **Over what period of time**?	Two months.	
	20 **Fatigue**?	Yes, I'm tired all the time.	✓
	21 **Numbness or tingling**?	No.	✓
	22 **Visual changes**?	No.	✓
Social Hx	23 What does your **diet** look like?	My husband likes a lot of pasta.	
(FED TACOS)	24 Do you **exercise**?	I try, but I'm too tired.	
	25 Do you **smoke**?	No.	✓
	26 Drink **alcohol**?	No.	✓
	27 Do you drink **caffeine**?	No.	✓
	28 **Occupation**?	I teach 5th grade.	✓
	29 Are you **sexually active**?	Yes	✓
	30 Do you use **protection**?	Yes. We use condoms.	✓
	31 Does your **partner have any symptoms**?	Like what?	
	32 Does he have any **discharge or burning**?	No.	
	33 When was the **FDLMP**?	Last Week	✓
Medical Hx	34 Do you have any medical conditions.	No.	✓
Allergies	35 Do you have any allergies?	No.	✓
Surg Hx	36 Have you had any surgeries?	No.	✓
Hosp Hx	37 Have you ever been hospitalized?	No.	✓
Family Hx	38 Medical conditions that run in the family?	Yes, both of my parents are diabetic.	✓
Medications	39 Are you on any medications?	No.	✓

Physical Examination ✓

	40	Informs patient that the physical exam is to begin and asks permission.		
	41	Rewashes hand before touching patient if candidate has recontaminated them.		
Eyes	42	Ophthalmoscopic examination	**No diabetic retinopathy noted b/l**	
	43	Right eye to right eye, left eye to left eye		
Neck	44	Inspection	**No masses, thyromegaly**	
	45	Palpation	**No thyromegaly**	
Cardiac	46	Auscultation performed on bare skin	**Reg rhythm w/o murmurs, rubs or gallop**	✓
	47	Areas: aortic, pulmonic, tricuspid, and mitral		
Respiratory	48	Auscultation performed on bare skin.	**Clear to auscultation**	✓
	49	Through complete inspiration and expiration		
	50	Symmetrically		
	51	At least 2 anterior levels, 1 lateral, and 3 posterior		
Abdominal	52	Helps patient with position changes.		✓
	53	Covers lower extremities with a sheet during the exam.		✓
	54	Inspection: Properly exposes the abdomen	**Obese**	✓
	55	Auscultation prior to palpation	**NABS without bruit**	✓
Vascular	56	Palpation of bilateral distal pulses	**2/4 upper and lower extremities**	
Neurologic	57	Sensory examination	**Intact**	
	58	Reflexes	**2/4 throughout**	
Assessment	59	Presents patient with a proposed diagnosis.	**Polyuria: Diabetes vs. UTI**	
Plan	60	MTHR: Office urine dip, urinalysis, labs, diet and exercise counseling, referral		
(MOTHRR)	61	Return plan: Devises and explains a follow-up plan with the patient.		
	62	Thanks the patient and asks if there are any questions.		

Humanistic Evaluation Y/N

Did the candidate present in a self-caring manner (e.g., hair control, clothing, cleanliness, aroma, etc.)?	
Did the candidate make periodic eye contact?	
Was the candidate's language clear and EASY to understand?	
Did the candidate have any substance in his or her mouth during the session?	
Did the candidate exhibit body language that would make you feel the candidate was communicating with you?	
Was the candidate enthusiastic?	
Did the candidate exhibit pride in his or her efforts?	
Did the candidate make any comment regarding your lifestyle (e.g., your work, family, activities, etc.)?	
Did the candidate express any humanistic statement recognizing your concerns?	
Did the candidate explain the medical problem and offer you a possible diagnosis?	
Did the candidate suggest a treatment plan that you could understand?	
Did the candidate inquire whether you might want to consult with family members or others about your visit?	
Did the candidate present as if he or she were a competent interviewer? Did the candidate ask you if you had any questions?	
Did the candidate thank you?	

Case 13

Patient Name:	Edward Amedus
Clinical Setting:	Emergency Room
CC:	A 72 y/o male presents with leg pain.

Vital Signs

Blood pressure:	148/88
Respirations:	12 per minute
Temperature:	100.6°F
Pulse:	84 bpm
Weight:	192 lbs
Height:	6'1"

NOTES:

Subjective

Objective

Assessment

Plan

CC: A 72 y/o male presents with leg pain.

History			✓
	1 Introduces self and explains role of provider.		✓
	2 Properly washes hands before touching the patient (15-sec wash and turns off with towel).		✓
	3 Opening question: What brings you in today?	My leg hurts.	✓
Chronology/ Onset	4 **When** did it first **start**?	I noticed it yesterday morning.	✓
	5 How has it **changed**?	The pain seems to be getting worse.	
	6 Did this ever happen **before**?	No.	✓
	7 Was there any **trauma**?	No.	
Description	8 **Where** is the pain?	It's my right calf.	✓
	9 **What is the intensity** on a scale of 1 to 10?	I'd say it was a 6.	✓
Exacerbation	10 What makes it **worse**?	It's worse when I'm walking on it.	✓
Remission	11 What make it **better**?	I took some Tylenol, but it didn't do much.	✓
Symptoms associated	12 **Swelling**?	It was last night when I went to bed.	
	13 **Redness**?	Yes.	
	14 **Warmth**?	Yes.	
	15 **Numbness or tingling**?	No.	
	16 **Fever or chills**?	No. I don't think so.	✓
	17 **Shortness of breath or chest pain**?	No.	✓
Social Hx	18 What does your **diet** look like?	I really watch it, lean meat and a lot of fruits.	
(FED TACOS)	19 Do you **exercise**?	Yes. I swim every day at the YMCA.	
	20 Have you **traveled** recently?	Yes, we just drove back from Florida.	✓
	21 Do you **smoke**?	No.	✓
	22 Do you drink **alcohol**?	No.	✓
	23 What is your **occupation**?	I'm a book reviewer.	✓
Medical Hx	24 Do you have any other **medical conditions**?	I have reflux.	✓
Allergies	25 Do you have any allergies?	No.	✓
Surg Hx	26 Have you had any surgeries?	No.	✓
Hosp Hx	27 Have you ever been hospitalized?	No.	✓
Family Hx	28 Medical conditions that run in the family?	Heart problems are a little prevalent.	✓
Medications	29 What **medications** are you on?	Ranitidine.	✓
	30 **What is the dose**?	75 mg.	✓
	31 How many times **per day**?	Once a day.	✓

Physical Examination ✓

			✓
	32 Informs patient that the physical exam is to begin and asks permission.		
	33 Rewashes hand before touching patient if candidate has recontaminated them.		
General	34 Assesses for **distress**.	**No distress**	
Vitals	35 Repeats BP with correct technique.	**152/90 right arm**	
	36 Appropriate size cuff		
	37 Applied correctly placing cuff on bare arm		
Neck	38 Auscultation for carotid bruit	**No bruit**	✓
Cardiac	39 Auscultation performed on bare skin	**Reg rhythm w/o murmur, rub, or gallop**	✓
	40 Areas: aortic, pulmonic, tricuspid, and mitral		
Respiratory	41 Auscultation performed on bare skin	**Clear to auscultation**	✓
	42 Through complete inspiration and expiration		
	43 Symmetrically		
	44 At least 2 anterior levels, 1 lateral, and 3 posterior		
Abdomen	45 Helps patient with position changes.		
	46 Covers lower extremities with a sheet during the exam.		
	47 Inspection: Properly exposes the abdomen	**Flat without masses**	
	48 Auscultation prior to palpation	**NABS. No bruits**	
	49 Palpation	**No masses or aortic aneurysm**	
Extremity	50 Inspection: Exposes bilateral lower extremities	**Erythema, 2+ edema right knee down**	✓
	51 Palpation: Compares bilaterally	**Increased warmth. Tenderness R calf**	✓
	52 Homans' sign: Rapid dorsiflexion of the foot	**Possible positive on the right**	✓
	53 Peripheral pulses	**Intact dorsal pedis and post tibialis**	✓
Assessment	54 Presents patient with a proposed diagnosis.	**DVT, elevated blood pressure**	✓
Plan	55 MTHR: Pain relief, imaging, laboratory analysis, leg elevation, consultation		✓
(MOTHRR)	56 Advises admission and DVT evaluation.		✓
	57 Thanks the patient and asks if there are any questions.		✓

Humanistic Evaluation Y/N

	Y/N
Did the candidate present in a self-caring manner (e.g., hair control, clothing, cleanliness, aroma, etc.)?	
Did the candidate make periodic eye contact?	
Was the candidate's language clear and EASY to understand?	
Did the candidate have any substance in his or her mouth during the session?	
Did the candidate exhibit body language that would make you feel the candidate was communicating with you?	
Was the candidate enthusiastic?	
Did the candidate exhibit pride in his or her efforts?	
Did the candidate make any comment regarding your lifestyle (e.g., your work, family, activities, etc.)?	
Did the candidate express any humanistic statement recognizing your concerns?	
Did the candidate explain the medical problem and offer you a possible diagnosis?	
Did the candidate suggest a treatment plan that you could understand?	
Did the candidate inquire whether you might want to consult with family members or others about your visit?	
Did the candidate present as if he or she were a competent interviewer?	
Did the candidate ask you if you had any questions?	
Did the candidate thank you?	

Case 14

Patient Name: Letzhavia Bebe
Clinical Setting: Family Practice Office
CC: A 25 y/o female presents for "fertility planning."

Vital Signs
Blood pressure: 108/72
Respirations: 12 per minute
Temperature: 98.6°F
Pulse: 70 bpm
Weight: 138 lbs
Height: 5'5"

NOTES:

Subjective

Objective

Assessment

Plan

CC: A 25 y/o female presents for "fertility planning."

History			✓
	1	Introduces self and explains role of provider.	✓
	2	Properly washes hands before touching the patient (15-sec wash and turns off with towel).	✓
	3	Opening question: What brings you in today?	I'm planning to become pregnant.	✓
Chronology/ Onset	4	**When** do you plan to become pregnant? Within the next few months.	✓
	5	Have you ever been **pregnant before**? No.	
Social Hx	6	What is your **diet** like? I think it's pretty balanced.	
(FED TACOS)	7	Do you **exercise**? I walk almost every day.	
	8	How far? About a half hour or more.	
	9	Do you **smoke**? Yes, but I plan to quit.	✓
	10	**How much** a day? Half a pack per day.	✓
	11	**How many years**? Three years or so.	✓
	12	Do you drink **alcohol**? A little.	✓
	13	**How much** a day? Not every day. A couple beers a week.	✓
	14	Do you drink **caffeine**? I drink three pops a day.	✓
	15	Do you use any **drugs**? No.	✓
	16	**Occupation**? I'm a manager at a grocery store.	✓
	17	Do they provide you with health insurance? Yes.	
	18	Are you **married**? Yes.	✓
	19	How long have you been married? Almost a year.	✓
	20	How does he feel about having a baby? I'm sure he'll be happy.	
	21	Have you told him you plan to get pregnant? It's popped up now and then.	
Medical Hx	22	Do you have any medical conditions? No.	✓
Ob/GYN Hx	23	When was your **first menses**? I was 11.	
	24	Are they **regular**? Like clockwork, every 28 days.	✓
	25	When was the **FDLMP**. Two weeks ago.	✓
	26	How old were you when you **first had sex**? Seventeen.	
	27	How many **partners**? Five.	
	28	History of **sexually transmitted diseases**? No.	
	29	**Last breast and pelvic exam**? About 6 months ago.	
	30	Was it normal? Yes.	
Allergies	31	Do you have any allergies? No.	✓
Surg Hx	32	Have you had any surgeries? I had my tonsils out when I was a kid.	✓
Hosp Hx	33	Have you ever been hospitalized? No.	✓
Family Hx	34	Medical conditions that run in the family? I have a brother with Down syndrome.	✓
Medications	35	Are you on any **medications**? I'm on the Pill, but I'm going to stop it.	✓

Physical Examination ✓

	36	Informs patient that the physical exam is to begin and asks permission.	
	37	Rewashes hand before touching patient if candidate has recontaminated them.	
HEENT	38	Inspection	**PERRLA, no pallor or lesions**
Neck	39	Palpation	**No thyromegaly or masses** ✓
Lymphatics	40	Palpation	**No lymphadenopathy** ✓
Respiratory	41	Auscultation performed on bare skin	**Clear to auscultation** ✓
	42	Through complete inspiration and expiration	
	43	Symmetrically	
	44	At least 2 anterior levels, 1 lateral, and 3 posterior	
Cardiac	45	Auscultation performed on bare skin	**RR without murmurs, rubs, gallops** ✓
	46	Areas: aortic, pulmonic, tricuspid, and mitral	
Abdomen	47	Helps patient to supine position.	
	48	Drapes lower extremities with sheet.	
	49	Inspection	**Rounded** ✓
	50	Auscultation prior to palpation	**Normoactive bowel sounds** ✓
	51	Palpation	**No masses or organomegaly** ✓
Breast	52	Advises SP that breast exam should be performed.	**Does not perform exam.**
Genitalia	53	Advises SP that pelvic exam should be performed.	**Does not perform exam.**
Extremities	54	Inspection	**No edema or cyanosis.**
	55	Palpation	**Peripheral pulses 2/4 throughout**
Assessment	56	Presents patient with at least one diagnosis.	**Fertility planning**
Plan	57	MTHR: Folic acid, diet, exercise, smoking/alcohol cessation, labs, referral	
(MOTHRR)	58	Social intervention: Offer to have husband come in for counseling/planning.	
	59	Education: Most patients become pregnant within 6 to 12 months of unprotected intercourse.	
	60	Return plan: Devises and explains a follow-up plan including breast and pelvic exams.	
	61	Thanks the patient and asks if there are any questions.	

Humanistic Evaluation Y/N

Did the candidate present in a self-caring manner (e.g., hair control, clothing, cleanliness, aroma, etc.)?	
Did the candidate make periodic eye contact?	
Was the candidate's language clear and EASY to understand?	
Did the candidate have any substance in his or her mouth during the session?	
Did the candidate exhibit body language that would make you feel the candidate was communicating with you?	
Was the candidate enthusiastic?	
Did the candidate exhibit pride in his or her efforts?	
Did the candidate make any comment regarding your lifestyle (e.g., your work, family, activities, etc.)?	
Did the candidate express any humanistic statement recognizing your concerns?	
Did the candidate explain the medical problem and offer you a possible diagnosis?	
Did the candidate suggest a treatment plan that you could understand?	
Did the candidate inquire whether you might want to consult with family members or others about your visit?	
Did the candidate present as if he or she were a competent interviewer?	
Did the candidate ask you if you had any questions?	
Did the candidate thank you?	

Patient Name: Hiram Tentson
Clinical Setting: Family Practice Office
CC: A 51 y/o AA male presents for evaluation of blood pressure.

Vital Signs
Blood pressure: 182/96
Respirations: 16 per minute
Temperature: 96.8°F
Pulse: 62 bpm
Weight: 242 lbs
Height: 6' 4"

NOTES:

Subjective

Objective

Assessment

Plan

CC: A 51 y/o AA male presents for evaluation of blood pressure.

History			✓
	1 Introduces self and explains role of provider.		✓
	2 Properly washes hands before touching the patient (15-sec wash and turns off with towel).		✓
	3 Opening question: What brings you in today?	I was told my blood pressure was up again.	✓
Chronology/ Onset	4 **When** were you told that?	Last week.	✓
	5 **Who** told you it was elevated?	A screener at the health fair.	✓
Duration	6 Did you ever have this **before**?	Yes.	✓
	7 When?	A couple of years ago.	✓
	8 Were you treated for it?	I was supposed to be, but I didn't refill it.	✓
	9 **How long ago** did you **run out of pills**?	About a year ago.	
	10 Do you remember the **name** of it?	No, some big long word.	✓
	11 **Why** did you **stop** taking it?	It made me feel tired.	✓
Symptoms associated	12 **Headaches**?	No.	
	13 **Palpitations/sweating**?	No.	✓
	14 **Weakness/polyuria**?	No.	
	15 **Claudication**?	No.	
	16 **Chest pain/dyspnea on exertion**?	No.	✓
	17 **Visual changes**?	No.	
	18 **Stress or anxiety**?	My work is kind of tough.	
	19 What is your **profession**?	I'm an editor.	✓
Social Hx	20 Do you use **salt** in your diet?	I like my salt.	
(FED TACOS)	21 Do you **exercise**?	No.	
	22 Do you **smoke**?	A little.	✓
	23 **How much** a day?	About a half pack.	✓
	24 **How many years**?	About 30 or so.	✓
	25 Do you drink **alcohol**?	No.	✓
	26 Do you drink **caffeine**?	About a pot of regular a day.	✓
	27 Do you use any **drugs**?	Are you crazy?	✓
Medical Hx	28 Do you have any medical conditions?	Just a runny nose from allergies.	✓
Allergies	29 Do you have any allergies?	Just to the environment.	✓
Surg Hx	30 Have you had any surgeries?	No.	✓
Hosp Hx	31 Have you ever been hospitalized?	No.	
Family Hx	32 Family Hx (i.e., htn, heart attack, or stroke)?	My parents died at 50 of the heart.	✓
Medications	33 Are you on any medications?	Sudafed for my allergies.	✓
	34 **How** many **milligrams**?	Two tablets at a time. I don't know the dose.	✓
	35 How **often**?	Two or 3 times a day when pollen is bad.	

Physical Examination ✓

	36	Informs patient that the physical exam is to begin and asks permission.	
	37	Rewashes hands before touching patient if candidate has recontaminated them.	
General	38	Inspection	**WDWN, NAD**
Vitals	39	Repeats BP in each arm.	**BP 176/96**
	40	Appropriate size cuff	
	41	Applied correctly placing cuff on bare arm	
Neck	42	Auscultation	**No bruit**
	43	Palpation	**No thyromegaly**
Eyes	44	Ophthalmoscopic exam	**No papilledema, hypertensive changes**
Cardiac	45	Inspection: Properly exposes the chest	**No heave or visible PMI**
	46	Auscultation performed on bare skin	**Reg rhythm w/o murmur, rub, or gallop**
	47	Areas: aortic, pulmonic, tricuspid, and mitral	
	48	Palpation for PMI	**Anterior axillary line 5th ICS**
Respiratory	49	Auscultation performed on bare skin	**Clear to auscultation**
	50	Through complete inspiration and expiration	
	51	Symmetrically	
	52	At least 2 anterior levels, 1 lateral, and 3 posterior	
Abdominal	53	Helps patient with position changes.	
	54	Covers lower extremities with a sheet during the exam.	
	55	Inspection: Properly exposes the abdomen	**No masses**
	56	Auscultation prior to palpation	**NABS without bruit**
	57	Palpation of size of abdominal aorta	**No pulsatile masses**
Vascular	58	Palpation	**Peripheral pulses 2/4 throughout**
Assessment	59	Presents patient with a proposed diagnosis.	**Hypertension**
Plan	60	MTHR: Antihypertensive, discontinue OTC medication, labs, smoking cessation	
(MOTHRR)	61	Return plan: Devises and explains a follow-up plan with the patient.	
	62	Thanks the patient and asks if there are any questions.	

Humanistic Evaluation Y/N

Did the candidate present in a self-caring manner (e.g., hair control, clothing, cleanliness, aroma, etc.)?	
Did the candidate make periodic eye contact?	
Was the candidate's language clear and EASY to understand?	
Did the candidate have any substance in his or her mouth during the session?	
Did the candidate exhibit body language that would make you feel the candidate was communicating with you?	
Was the candidate enthusiastic?	
Did the candidate exhibit pride in his or her efforts?	
Did the candidate make any comment regarding your lifestyle (e.g., your work, family, activities, etc.)?	
Did the candidate express any humanistic statement recognizing your concerns?	
Did the candidate explain the medical problem and offer you a possible diagnosis?	
Did the candidate suggest a treatment plan that you could understand?	
Did the candidate inquire whether you might want to consult with family members or others about your visit?	
Did the candidate present as if he or she were a competent interviewer?	
Did the candidate ask you if you had any questions?	
Did the candidate thank you?	

Case 16

Patient Name:	Chuckie Yupp
Clinical Setting:	Family Practice Office
CC:	A 4-month-old male presents with his mother for "spitting up."

Vital Signs

Blood pressure:	80/50
Respirations:	35 per minute
Temperature:	98.4°F
Pulse:	120 bpm
Weight:	13 lbs
Height:	22 1/2 inches

NOTES:

Subjective

Objective

Assessment

Plan

CC: A 4-month-old male presents with his mother for "spitting up."

History ✓

	1	Introduces self and explains role of provider.		
	2	Properly washes hands before touching the patient (15-sec wash and turns off with towel).		
	3	Opening question: What brings you in today?	The baby is spitting up all the time.	✓
Chronology/Onset	4	**When** did this start?	He has always spit up, ever since he was born.	✓
	5	**How often** does it happen?	Several times a day.	✓
	6	**Does it happen any particular times**?	Usually after feeding him his bottle.	✓
Description	7	Could you **describe what comes up**?	It's his formula.	✓
	8	**Does it dribble or shoot out of his mouth**?	Usually it dribbles. Occasionally it shoots.	✓
Exacerbation	9	Does anything make it **worse**?	If he drinks a whole bottle.	✓
Remission	10	What makes it **better**?	Feeding him smaller bottles.	✓
Symptoms associated	11	**Weight loss?**	He's put on half a pound since the last visit.	✓
	12	**Difficulty breathing?**	No.	✓
	13	**Pain?**	No.	
	14	**Irritability?**	No.	✓
	15	**Cough?**	No.	✓
	16	**Turn blue or dusky?**	No.	✓
	17	**Spit up blood?**	No.	
	18	**Constipation or diarrhea?**	He strains sometimes.	✓
	19	**Fever?**	No.	✓
Social Hx	20	Do you or does anyone in the house **smoke**?	Yes, his father does.	
Medical Hx	21	Does he have any medical conditions?	No.	✓
Allergies	22	Does he have any allergies?	No.	✓
Surg Hx	23	Has he had any surgeries?	No.	✓
Hosp Hx	24	Has he ever been hospitalized?	No.	✓
Family Hx	25	Medical conditions that run in the family?	My husband has bad reflux.	✓
Medications	26	Is he on any medications?	No.	✓

Physical Examination   ✓

	27	Informs patient that the physical exam is to begin and asks permission.	
	28	Rewashes hands before touching patient if candidate has recontaminated them.	
General	29	Inspection	**Well nourished/developed. No distress**
Skin	30	Inspection	**No rashes or lesions**
	31	Palpation	**Warm and dry**
	32	Turgor	**Intact**
Head	33	Inspection	**Normocephalic. Fontanelles flat**
	34	Palpation	**Fontanelles are open and soft.**
Nose	35	Inspection	**Without deformity of discharge**
Throat	36	Inspection with tongue blade and light source	**Pink without injection. No deformity** ✓
	37	Gag reflex	**Intact** ✓
Neck	38	Inspection	**Supple**
Cardiac	39	Inspection: Properly exposes the chest	**No heave or visible PMI** ✓
	40	Auscultation performed on bare skin	**Reg rhythm w/o murmur, rub, or gallop** ✓
	41	Areas: aortic, pulmonic, tricuspid, and mitral	
Respiratory	42	Auscultation performed on bare skin	**Clear to auscultation** ✓
	43	Through complete inspiration and expiration	
	44	Symmetrically	
	45	At least 2 anterior levels, 1 lateral, and 3 posterior	
Abdominal	46	Inspection: Properly exposes the abdomen	**Rounded** ✓
	47	Auscultation prior to palpation	**NABS** ✓
	48	Palpation	**No masses, organomegaly** ✓
Assessment	49	Presents patient with a proposed diagnosis.	**Uncomplicated reflux**
Plan	50	MTHR: Avoid overfeeding and tobacco smoke. Upright for feedings	
(MOTHRR)	51	Return plan: Devises and explains a follow-up plan with the patient.	
	52	Thanks the mother and asks if there are any questions.	

Humanistic Evaluation   Y/N

Did the candidate present in a self-caring manner (e.g., hair control, clothing, cleanliness, aroma, etc.)?	
Did the candidate make periodic eye contact?	
Was the candidate's language clear and EASY to understand?	
Did the candidate have any substance in his or her mouth during the session?	
Did the candidate exhibit body language that would make you feel the candidate was communicating with you?	
Was the candidate enthusiastic?	
Did the candidate exhibit pride in his or her efforts?	
Did the candidate make any comment regarding your lifestyle (e.g., your work, family, activities, etc.)?	
Did the candidate express any humanistic statement recognizing your concerns?	
Did the candidate explain the medical problem and offer you a possible diagnosis?	
Did the candidate suggest a treatment plan that you could understand?	
Did the candidate inquire whether you might want to consult with family members or others about your visit?	
Did the candidate present as if he or she were a competent interviewer?	
Did the candidate ask you if you had any questions?	
Did the candidate thank you?	

Patient Name: Emmanuel Iskus
Clinical Setting: Primary Care Outpatient Office Visit
CC: A 30 y/o male presents c/o knee pain.

Vital Signs
Blood pressure: 120/72
Respirations: 12 per minute
Temperature: 98.8°F
Pulse: 62 bpm
Weight: 182 lbs
Height: 6'3"

NOTES:

Subjective

Objective

Assessment

Plan

CC: A 30 y/o male presents c/o knee pain.

History			✓
	1 Introduces self and explains role of provider.		✓
	2 Properly washes hands before touching the patient (15-sec wash and turns off with towel).		✓
	3 Opening question: What brings you in today?	I hurt my right knee.	✓
Chronology/ Onset	4 **How** did you hurt it?	Playing paintball.	✓
	5 **When** did it happen?	Last night.	✓
	6 Did you hurt this knee **before**?	Yes.	✓
	7 **When**?	Last year playing basketball.	✓
	8 **Prior diagnosis/How was it treated?**	They wrapped it and sent me to therapy.	✓
Description/	9 **Describe** how it happened.	I stepped in a hole and my leg buckled.	✓
Duration	10 **Where** is the pain?	Along the inside.	
Intensity	11 **Intensity** on a scale of 1 to 10?	About a 5.	✓
Exacerbation	12 What makes it **worse**?	Standing on it.	✓
Remission	13 What makes it **better**?	Ice helped a little.	✓
Symptoms associated	14 Any **bruising**?	Yes.	
	15 Any **swelling**?	There was some last night.	
	16 Is the **range of motion** limited?	I can't bend or straighten it the whole way.	
	17 Does the knee **click or lock**?	I do hear a popping.	
	18 **Numbness or tingling**?	No.	✓
Social Hx	19 Do you **exercise**?	At least an hour a day.	✓
(FED TACOS)	20 Do you **smoke or use tobacco**?	No.	✓
	21 Do you drink **alcohol**?	No.	✓
	22 What is your **occupation**?	I'm a high school football coach.	✓
Medical Hx	23 Do you have any medical conditions?	I have asthma.	✓
Allergies	24 Do you have any allergies?	No.	✓
Surgical Hx	25 Have you had any surgeries?	Yes.	✓
	26 What was that?	They scoped the same knee.	✓
	27 Did they find anything?	They shaved a little off the meniscus.	✓
Hosp Hx	28 Have you ever been hospitalized?	No.	✓
Family Hx	29 Medical conditions that run in the family?	High cholesterol.	✓
Medications	30 Are you on any medications?	Only a puffer as needed.	✓
	31 What is the name of it?	Albuterol.	✓
	32 How often do you need it?	A couple of times a year, I guess.	✓

Physical Examination   ✓

	33	Informs patient that the physical exam is to begin and asks permission.		
	34	Rewashes hands before touching patient if candidate has recontaminated them.		
MS	35	Covers patient with a sheet from waist down.		
	36	Raises sheet to expose bilateral lower extremities.		
	37	Inspection of right knee	**Ecchymosis R medial tibial plateau**	✓
	38	Comparison to left knee		✓
	39	Active range of motion	**Limited extension and flexion Right**	✓
	40	Passive range of motion	**Limited extension because of pain**	✓
	41	Palpation	**Tenderness R lat joint space**	✓
Position Change	42	Assists patient to supine position.		✓
Special Testing	43	Drawer testing	**Negative**	
	44	Varus/valgus stress tests	**Negative**	✓
	45	McMurray's test	**Positive**	✓
Neurologic	46	Sensory exam light touch or sharp vs. dull	**Intact**	
Vascular	47	Peripheral pulses	**Intact**	
Gait	48	Helps patient with position change to standing.		
	49	Assesses gait.	**Patient walks with limp on right.**	
Assessment	50	Presents patient with a proposed diagnosis.	**Meniscal injury**	✓
Plan	51	MTHR: Pain control, testing (radiograph), holistic (RICE), referral (PT)		
(MOTHRR)	52	Explains and offers OMM.		✓
	53	Performs OMM appropriately (no HVLA).		✓
	54	Return plan: Devises and explains a follow-up plan with the patient.		
	55	Thanks the patient and asks if there are any questions.		

Humanistic Evaluation   Y/N

Did the candidate present in a self-caring manner (e.g., hair control, clothing, cleanliness, aroma, etc.)?	
Did the candidate make periodic eye contact?	
Was the candidate's language clear and EASY to understand?	
Did the candidate have any substance in his or her mouth during the session?	
Did the candidate exhibit body language that would make you feel the candidate was communicating with you?	
Was the candidate enthusiastic?	
Did the candidate exhibit pride in his or her efforts?	
Did the candidate make any comment regarding your lifestyle (e.g., your work, family, activities, etc.)?	
Did the candidate express any humanistic statement recognizing your concerns?	
Did the candidate explain the medical problem and offer you a possible diagnosis?	
Did the candidate suggest a treatment plan that you could understand?	
Did the candidate inquire whether you might want to consult with family members or others about your visit?	
Did the candidate present as if he or she were a competent interviewer?	
Did the candidate ask you if you had any questions?	
Did the candidate thank you?	

Case 18

Patient Name:	Lucy Flemming
Clinical Setting:	Family Practice Office
CC:	A 62 y/o female presents for "coughing all the time."

Vital Signs

Blood pressure:	174/95
Respirations:	16 per minute
Temperature:	99.2°F
Pulse:	92 bpm
Weight:	125 lbs
Height	5' 4"

NOTES:

Subjective

Objective

Assessment

Plan

CC: A 62 y/o female presents for "coughing all the time."

History			✓
	1	Introduces self and explains role of provider.	
	2	Properly washes hands before touching the patient (15-sec wash and turns off with towel).	✓
	3	Opening question: What brings you in today?	I can't get rid of this cough.	✓
Chronology/ Onset	4	**When** did this start?	About 4 months ago.	✓
	5	Did you ever have this **before**?	No.	✓
	6	**How often** does it happen?	I'm coughing all the time.	✓
	7	What are you **doing** when it happens?	I can be doing anything.	✓
Description	8	Could you **describe the cough**?	It used to be dry, but now it's heavy.	✓
	9	Are you **bringing anything up**?	Yes.	✓
	10	What does it look like?	It used to be clear, but now it's bloody.	✓
Exacerbation	11	Does anything make it **worse**?	Exerting myself, like walking.	✓
Remission	12	What makes it **better**?	Resting.	✓
Symptoms associated	13	Do you have any pain?	Just from coughing.	✓
	14	Where is the pain?	*Holds right rib cage*	✓
	15	On a scale from 0 to 10?	A 6.	
	16	**Shortness of breath?**	Sometimes during coughing fits.	✓
	17	**Tired?**	I'm always tired.	✓
	18	**Weight lost?**	Oh, yes.	✓
	19	How much weight?	Twenty pounds.	✓
	20	Over what period of time?	Maybe 3 months.	✓
	21	**Bone pain?**	I have a little arthritis.	✓
	22	**Fever?**	No.	✓
	23	**Night sweats?**	I do wake up a little sweaty.	
Social Hx	24	Do you **smoke**?	I quit last year.	✓
(FED TACOS)	25	**How much** a day?	Two packs.	✓
	26	**How many years?**	Since I was 14.	✓
	27	Do you drink **alcohol**?	No.	✓
	28	Do you drink **caffeine**?	Two cups of coffee each morning.	✓
	29	What is your **occupation**?	I'm a house wife.	✓
Medical Hx	30	Do you have any medical conditions?	High blood pressure.	✓
Allergies	31	Do you have any allergies?	No.	✓
Surg Hx	32	Have you had any surgeries?	I had a hysterectomy at 40.	✓
Hosp Hx	33	Have you ever been hospitalized?	I had pneumonia a few months ago.	✓
Family Hx	34	Medical conditions that run in the family?	My father had kidney cancer.	✓
Medications	35	Are you on any medications?	Metoprolol.	✓
	36	How many pills a day?	One in the morning and one at night.	✓
	37	How many milligrams?	I'm not sure.	✓

Physical Examination ✓

	38	Informs patient that the physical exam is to begin and asks permission.	
	39	Rewashes hand before touching patient if candidate has recontaminated them.	
Vitals	40	Repeats the blood pressure with correct technique. **160/85**	
	41	Appropriate size cuff, applied correctly	
Throat	42	Inspection with tongue blade and light source	**Pink without erythema or exudate** ✓
Neck	43	Inspection	**Symmetrical** ✓
	44	Palpation	**Without masses** ✓
Lymphatics	45	Cervical and axillary nodes	**Right supraclavicular 2-cm node** ✓
Respiratory	46	Inspection: Properly exposes the chest	**Crackles right middle lobe** ✓
	47	Auscultation performed on bare skin	**Wheezing right middle/lower lobes** ✓
	48	Through complete inspiration and expiration	✓
	49	Symmetrically	✓
	50	At least 2 anterior levels, 1 lateral, and 3 posterior	✓
	51	Palpation	**Nontender to palpation**
Cardiac	52	Auscultation performed on bare skin	**RR without murmurs, rubs, or gallop** ✓
	53	Areas: aortic, pulmonic, tricuspid, and mitral	✓
Abdominal	54	Drapes lower extremities with sheet.	
	55	Helps patient to supine position.	
	56	Inspection: Exposes abdomen leaving sheet intact	
	57	Auscultation	**Normoactive bowel sounds**
	58	Palpation watching facial expression	**Nontender without masses**
	59	Helps patient to seated position.	
Assessment	60	Presents patient with a proposed diagnosis.	**May include possible lung cancer** ✓
Plan	61	MTHR: Antibiotic, imaging, smoking cessation, referral	
(MOTHRR)	62	Return plan: Devises and explains a follow-up plan with the patient.	
	63	Thanks the patient and asks if there are any questions.	

Humanistic Evaluation Y/N

Did the candidate present in a self-caring manner (e.g., hair control, clothing, cleanliness, aroma, etc.)?	
Did the candidate make periodic eye contact?	
Was the candidate's language clear and EASY to understand?	
Did the candidate have any substance in his or her mouth during the session?	
Did the candidate exhibit body language that would make you feel the candidate was communicating with you?	
Was the candidate enthusiastic?	
Did the candidate exhibit pride in his or her efforts?	
Did the candidate make any comment regarding your lifestyle (e.g., your work, family, activities, etc.)?	
Did the candidate express any humanistic statement recognizing your concerns?	
Did the candidate explain the medical problem and offer you a possible diagnosis?	
Did the candidate suggest a treatment plan that you could understand?	
Did the candidate inquire whether you might want to consult with family members or others about your visit?	
Did the candidate present as if he or she were a competent interviewer?	
Did the candidate ask you if you had any questions?	
Did the candidate thank you?	

Patient Name: Betty B. Karfle
Clinical Setting: Emergency Room
CC: A 20 y/o female presents with "My head hurts."

Vital Signs
Blood pressure: 120/64
Respirations: 16 per minute
Temperature: 102°F
Pulse: 112 bpm
Weight: 136 lbs
Height: 5' 5"

NOTES:

Subjective

Objective

Assessment

Plan

CC: A 20 y/o female presents with "My head hurts."

History			✓
	1	Introduces self and explains role of provider.	
	2	Properly washes hands before touching the patient (15-sec wash and turns off with towel).	✓
	3	Opening question: What brings you in today?	My head hurts.	✓
Chronology/ Onset	4	**When** did this start?	A day or two ago.	✓
	5	Did you ever have this **before**?	No.	✓
	6	Did it come on **suddenly** or **gradually**?	Gradually.	
Description	7	Could you **describe it**?	It's a really bad pressure feeling.	✓
	8	**Where** does it hurt?	My whole head and neck hurt.	✓
Duration	9	Is it **constant** or does it **come and go**?	Constant.	✓
Intensity	10	On a **scale** from 0 to 10?	10.	✓
Exacerbation	11	Does anything make it **worse**?	Moving my head.	✓
Remission	12	What makes it **better**?	Nothing.	✓
Symptoms associated	13	**Recent cold/URI symptoms?**	Yes, for about a week.	
	14	**Fever?**	I feel hot.	✓
	15	**Nausea or vomiting?**	I'm nauseated, but I haven't vomited.	✓
	16	**Confusion?**	I couldn't think right in class today.	✓
	17	**Stiff neck?**	Yes.	✓
	18	**Rash?**	No.	
	19	**Photophobia?**	Yes. The lights really bother my eyes.	✓
Social Hx	20	Do you use any **drugs**?	No.	
(FED TACOS)	21	Do you **smoke**?	No.	✓
	22	Do you drink **alcohol**?	No.	✓
	23	What is your **occupation**?	I go to Gannon University.	✓
Medical Hx	24	Do you have any medical conditions?	No.	✓
Allergies	25	Do you have any allergies?	No.	✓
Surgical Hx	26	Have you had any surgeries?	No.	✓
Hosp Hx	27	Have you ever been hospitalized?	No.	✓
Family Hx	28	Contacts with similar complaints?	Not that I know of.	✓
Medications	29	Are you on any medications?	I'm supposed to be.	✓
	30	Did you have immunizations for meningitis?	No.	

Physical Examination ✓

	31	Informs patient that the physical exam is to begin and asks permission.	
	32	Rewashes hand before touching patient if candidate has recontaminated them.	
Skin	33	Inspection	**No rash**
Head	34	Inspection/Palpation	**NCAT. Nontender**
Face	35	Cranial nerve VII	**Facial symmetry. Can close eyes**
	36	Cranial nerve V	**Masseter muscles intact**
Eyes	37	Inspection: CNIII, IV, and VI	**Extraocular movements intact**
	38	Pupillary reflex: CNII and CNIII	**PERRLA**
	39	Ophthalmoscopic examination	**Papilledema**
Throat	40	Cranial nerve X—have patient say "ah"	**Uvula rises midline**
	41	Cranial nerve XII—have patient stick out tongue	**No deviation**
Neck	42	Inspection	**No masses. Patient holding head still**
	43	Active range of motion	**Decreased in all fields**
	44	Palpation	**Nuchal rigidity**
	45	Kerning's or Brudzinski's	**Causes extreme pain**
Respiratory	46	Auscultation performed on bare skin	**Clear to auscultation**
	47	Through complete inspiration and expiration	
	48	Symmetrically	
	49	At least 2 anterior levels, 1 lateral, and 3 posterior	
Cardiac	50	Auscultation performed on bare skin	**RR without murmurs, rubs, or gallop**
	51	Areas: aortic, pulmonic, tricuspid, and mitral	
Neurologic	52	Motor strength testing with bilateral comparison	**5/5 throughout**
	53	Reflexes	**2/4 throughout**
	54	Babinski's exam	**Equivocal**
Assessment	55	Presents patient with a proposed diagnosis.	**Meningitis**
Plan	56	MTHR: Admission, stat imaging, labs, holistic (informs family), ID, and neuro consultation	
(MOTHRR)	57	Thanks the patient and asks if there are any questions.	

Humanistic Evaluation Y/N

Did the candidate present in a self-caring manner (e.g., hair control, clothing, cleanliness, aroma, etc.)?	
Did the candidate make periodic eye contact?	
Was the candidate's language clear and EASY to understand?	
Did the candidate have any substance in his or her mouth during the session?	
Did the candidate exhibit body language that would make you feel the candidate was communicating with you?	
Was the candidate enthusiastic?	
Did the candidate exhibit pride in his or her efforts?	
Did the candidate make any comment regarding your lifestyle (e.g., your work, family, activities, etc.)?	
Did the candidate express any humanistic statement recognizing your concerns?	
Did the candidate explain the medical problem and offer you a possible diagnosis?	
Did the candidate suggest a treatment plan that you could understand?	
Did the candidate inquire whether you might want to consult with family members or others about your visit?	
Did the candidate present as if he or she were a competent interviewer?	
Did the candidate ask you if you had any questions?	
Did the candidate thank you?	

Patient Name: Junie Laturel
Clinical Setting: Family Practice Outpatient Office Visit
CC: An 18 y/o female presents with a headache.

Vital Signs
Blood pressure: 110/60
Respirations: 16 per minute
Temperature: 98.0°F
Pulse: 92 bpm
Weight: 136 lbs
Height: 5'5"

NOTES:

Subjective

Objective

Assessment

Plan

CC: An 18 y/o female presents with a headache.

History			✓
	1 Introduces self and explains role of provider.		✓
	2 Properly washes hands before touching the patient (15-sec wash and turns off with towel).		✓
	3 Opening question: What brings you in today?	I have a headache.	✓
Chronology/ Onset	4 When did it **start**?	Well, this one started about 2 days ago.	✓
	5 Was the onset **sudden** or **gradual**?	They come on gradually.	
	6 **How often** do they occur?	I use to get them once a month, now I get one once a week.	✓
	7 When did you **first start getting them**?	About 2 or 3 years ago.	✓
	8 Can you tell they are **coming on**?	I see a fuzzy bright spot that gets bigger and bigger. Then, the headache starts.	✓
	9 What are you **doing at onset**?	They can happen any time.	
	10 **Triggers** (foods, stress, fatigue)?	Not that I know of.	
Description	11 **Describe** the headaches.	It's a pounding in my head.	✓
	12 **Location**?	They're always on the right side.	✓
Intensity	13 How severe is it, on a scale from **1 to 10**?	They can go up to a 10.	✓
Exacerbation	14 What makes it **worse**?	Bright lights.	✓
Remission	15 What makes it **better**?	I take ibuprofen and go to bed.	✓
Symptoms associated	16 **Nausea**?	Yes, after it starts, I feel like I want to vomit.	✓
	17 **Numbness/tingling/weakness**?	No.	✓
	18 **Depression or anxiety**?	These headaches stress me out.	
	19 **Fever or chills**?	No.	✓
	20 **Toothaches**?	No.	
	21 **Earaches**?	They get plugged up now and then.	
	22 **Sinus congestion**?	Only when my allergies act up.	
Social Hx	23 What does your **diet** look like?	It's not so good. I live for chocolate.	
(FED TACOS)	24 Do you **exercise**?	I play a lot of sports.	
	25 Do you **smoke**?	No.	✓
	26 Do you drink **alcohol**?	No.	✓
	27 Do you use any **drugs**?	No.	✓
	28 What is your **occupation**?	I'm in high school and work a burger place.	✓
Medical Hx	29 Do you have any medical conditions?	No.	✓
	30 History of **head trauma**?	No.	
Allergies	31 Do you have any allergies?	Just seasonal.	✓
Surgical Hx	32 Have you had any surgeries?	No.	✓
Hosp Hx	33 Have you ever been hospitalized?	No.	✓
Family Hx	34 Any medical conditions that run in the family?	Not that I know of.	✓
Medications	35 Are you on any medications?	Just birth control pills.	✓
FDLNMP	36 When was the FDLMP?	A couple of weeks ago.	✓

Physical Examination ✓

	37	Informs patient that the physical exam is to begin and asks permission.	
	38	Rewashes hand before touching patient if candidate has recontaminated them.	
Head	39	Inspection	**NCAT without lesions**
	40	Palpation	**Nontender to palpation**
Sinuses	41	Palpation, percussion	**Nontender**
Eyes	42	Ophthalmoscopic examination	**Cup:disc ratio 1:2 with sharp margins**
Nose	43	Inspection	**No exudate, edema, masses**
Ears	44	Inspection	**TM's gray bilaterally**
Mouth/throat	45	Inspection	**Teeth in good repair, no lesions, moist**
Neck	46	Inspection	**Symmetrical, no masses**
	47	Palpation	**Tissue texture changes T1-4 right**
Respiratory	48	Auscultation performed on bare skin	**Clear to auscultation**
	49	Through complete inspiration and expiration	
	50	Symmetrically	
	51	At least 2 anterior levels, 1 lateral, and 3 posterior	
Cardiac	52	Auscultation performed on bare skin	**RR without murmurs, rubs, or gallop**
	53	Areas: aortic, pulmonic, tricuspid, and mitral	
Neurologic	54	Motor strength testing with bilateral comparison	**5/5 throughout**
	55	Reflexes	**2/4 throughout**
Assessment	56	Presents patient with a proposed diagnosis.	**Migraine**
Plan	57	MTHR: Medication, headache log, trigger identification, consider imaging	
(MOTHRR)	58	Explains and offers OMM.	
	59	Performs OMM appropriately (no HVLA).	
	60	Return plan: Devises and explains a follow-up plan with the patient.	
	61	Thanks the patient and asks if there are any questions.	

Humanistic Evaluation Y/N

Did the candidate present in a self-caring manner (e.g., hair control, clothing, cleanliness, aroma, etc.)?	
Did the candidate make periodic eye contact?	
Was the candidate's language clear and EASY to understand?	
Did the candidate have any substance in his or her mouth during the session?	
Did the candidate exhibit body language that would make you feel the candidate was communicating with you?	
Was the candidate enthusiastic?	
Did the candidate exhibit pride in his or her efforts?	
Did the candidate make any comment regarding your lifestyle (e.g., your work, family, activities, etc.)?	
Did the candidate express any humanistic statement recognizing your concerns?	
Did the candidate explain the medical problem and offer you a possible diagnosis?	
Did the candidate suggest a treatment plan that you could understand?	
Did the candidate inquire whether you might want to consult with family members or others about your visit?	
Did the candidate present as if he or she were a competent interviewer?	
Did the candidate ask you if you had any questions?	
Did the candidate thank you?	

Case 21

Patient Name:	Nneka Soore
Clinical Setting:	Family Practice Outpatient Office Visit
CC:	A 49 y/o female presents with neck pain.

Vital Signs

Blood pressure:	158/88
Respirations:	14 per minute
Temperature:	98.4°F
Pulse:	72 bpm
Weight:	156 lbs
Height:	5' 3"

NOTES:

Subjective

Objective

Assessment

Plan

CC: A 49 y/o female presents with neck pain.

History			✓
	1	Introduces self and explains role of provider.	
	2	Properly washes hands before touching the patient (15-sec wash and turns off with towel).	
	3	Opening question: What brings you in today?	My neck hurts.	
Chronology/ Onset	4	**When** did it happen?	I just woke up like this today.	
	5	Have you ever had this **before**?	Yes, it acts up now and then.	
Description/ Duration	6	**Describe** the pain.	It's just tight and achy.	
	7	**Where** is the pain?	Right here. (*Grabs R superior trapezius*)	
Intensity	8	Intensity on a scale of 1 to 10?	I'd say it's a 7.	
Exacerbation	9	What makes it **worse**?	Moving my head too fast.	
Remission	10	What makes it **better**?	If I massage it.	
Symptoms associated	11	Any **trauma**?	I just must have slept on it wrong.	
	12	Any **swelling, redness, or bruising**?	No.	
	13	Is the **range of motion** limited?	Yes, I can't turn my head to the left.	
	14	**Numbness or weakness** of the arms?	No.	
	15	**Fever, chills, photophobia?**	No.	
Social Hx	16	Do you **exercise**?	I chase three grandkids around.	
(FED TACOS)	17	Do you **smoke**?	No.	
	18	Do you drink **alcohol**?	Yes.	
	19	**How much** a day?	A couple drinks a month.	
	20	Do you drink **caffeine**?	Two cups of coffee in the morning.	
	21	What is your **occupation**?	I do medical transcription.	
Medical Hx	22	Do you have any medical conditions?	I had fibroids.	
Allergies	23	Do you have any allergies?	No.	
Surg Hx	24	Have you had any surgeries?	When they took my uterus out.	
Hosp Hx	25	Have you ever been hospitalized?	Just for that surgery.	
Family Hx	26	Medical conditions that run in the family?	Diabetes runs in the family.	
	27	Any contacts with similar complaints?	No.	
Medications	28	Are you on any medications?	I just take a vitamin.	

Physical Examination ✓

	29	Informs patient that the physical exam is to begin and asks permission.	
	30	Rewashes hands before touching patient if candidate has recontaminated them.	
Vitals	31	Repeats BP with correct technique.	**BP 156/86**
	32	Appropriate size cuff	
	33	Applied correctly, placing cuff on bare arm	
Head	34	Inspection	**NCAT**
Neck	35	Inspection	**Symmetrical, no masses, erythema, edema**
	36	Range of motion	**Range of motion limited by pain with rotation or side bending to the left**
	37	Palpation	**Increased warmth, bogginess, tender at C5 transverse process, C5 RrSr**
Lymphatic	38	Cervical, axillary	**No lymphadenopathy**
Respiratory	39	Auscultation performed on bare skin	**Clear to auscultation**
	40	Through complete inspiration and expiration	
	41	Symmetrically	
	42	At least 2 anterior levels, 1 lateral, and 3 posterior	
Cardiac	43	Auscultation performed on bare skin	**RR without murmurs, rubs, gallops**
	44	Areas: aortic, pulmonic, tricuspid, and mitral	
Assessment	45	Presents patient with a proposed diagnosis.	**Cervical somatic dysfunction**
Plan	46	MTHR: Pain control, consider imaging, holistic (RICE), BP follow-up	
(MOTHRR)	47	Explains and offers OMM.	
	48	Performs OMM appropriately (no HVLA).	
	49	Return plan: Devises and explains a follow-up plan with the patient.	
	50	Thanks the patient and asks if there are any questions.	

Humanistic Evaluation Y/N

Did the candidate present in a self-caring manner (e.g., hair control, clothing, cleanliness, aroma, etc.)?	
Did the candidate make periodic eye contact?	
Was the candidate's language clear and EASY to understand?	
Did the candidate have any substance in his or her mouth during the session?	
Did the candidate exhibit body language that would make you feel the candidate was communicating with you?	
Was the candidate enthusiastic?	
Did the candidate exhibit pride in his or her efforts?	
Did the candidate make any comment regarding your lifestyle (e.g., your work, family, activities, etc.)?	
Did the candidate express any humanistic statement recognizing your concerns?	
Did the candidate explain the medical problem and offer you a possible diagnosis?	
Did the candidate suggest a treatment plan that you could understand?	
Did the candidate inquire whether you might want to consult with family members or others about your visit?	
Did the candidate present as if he or she were a competent interviewer?	
Did the candidate ask you if you had any questions?	
Did the candidate thank you?	

Case 22

Patient Name: Sid Koppe
Clinical Setting: Family Practice Office
CC: A 68 y/o male presents for "lightheadedness."

Vital Signs
Blood pressure: 103/80
Respirations: 16 per minute
Temperature: 98.8°F
Pulse: 72 bpm
Weight: 185 lbs
Height: 5'11"

NOTES:

Subjective

Objective

Assessment

Plan

CC: A 68 y/o male presents for "lightheadedness."

History			✓
	1 Introduces self and explains role of provider.		
	2 Properly washes hands before touching the patient (15-sec wash and turns off with towel).		
	3 Opening question: What brings you in today?	I get lightheaded when I stand up.	
Chronology/ Onset	4 **When** did this start?	About 2 weeks ago.	
	5 Did you ever have this **before**?	No.	
	6 **How often** does it happen?	Every time I get up from lying or sitting.	
	7 What are you **doing** when it happens?	Changing positions.	
	8 Does it come on **suddenly** or **gradually**?	Suddenly.	
Description Duration	9 Could you **describe it**?	When I stand up, I get lightheaded and have to wait a few seconds before I feel normal again.	
	10 **How long does it last** when it happens?	Less than a minute.	
Intensity	11 Have you **fallen**?	No.	
Exacerbation	12 Does anything make it **worse**?	It seems worse in the morning.	
Remission	13 What makes it **better**?	Nothing.	
Symptoms associated	14 **Weakness or fatigue?**	Yes, when I bend down to pick up my granddaughter it feels like my legs are going to give out.	
	15 **Difficulty concentrating?**	Not that I have noticed.	
	16 **Blacked out or lost consciousness?**	No.	
	17 **Heart racing?**	Yes, for a few minutes each time I change positions.	
	18 **Blurred vision?**	No.	
	19 **Shortness of breath?**	No.	
	20 **Change in your stools or dark tarry stools?**	No.	
Social Hx	21 What does your **diet** look like?	I watch the fats.	
(FED TACOS)	22 Do you **exercise**?	I push-mow my grass.	
	23 Do you **smoke**?	No.	
	24 Do you drink **alcohol**?	No.	
	25 What is your **occupation**?	I'm retired from the military.	
Medical Hx	26 Do you have any other **medical conditions**?	I just started taking medicine for high blood pressure.	
Allergies	27 Do you have any allergies?	No.	
Surgical Hx	28 Have you had any surgeries?	No.	
Hosp Hx	29 Have you ever been hospitalized?	No.	
Family Hx	30 Medical conditions that run in the family?	My father died in his 60s of a heart attack.	
Medications	31 Are you on any medications?	Hydrochlorothiazide.	
	32 How many times a day?	Once.	
	33 How many milligrams?	50 mg.	

Physical Examination   ✓

	34	Informs patient that the physical exam is to begin and asks permission.	
	35	Rewashes hands before touching patient if candidate has recontaminated them.	
Vitals	36	Performs orthostatic blood pressures.	**Lying 130/80, sit 120/72, stand 100/58**
Skin	37	Inspection	**Pale**
	38	Palpation	**Cool**
	39	Turgor	**Without tenting**
Neck	40	Auscultation of carotids prior to palpation	**Without bruits**
	41	Palpation of carotids	**2/4. Does not reproduce symptoms**
Cardiac	42	Inspection: Properly exposes the chest	**No heave or visible PMI**
	43	Auscultation performed on bare skin	**Reg rhythm w/o murmur, rub, or gallop**
	44	Palpation for PMI	**5th ICS 5 cm from sternal border**
Respiratory	45	Auscultation performed on bare skin	**Clear to auscultation**
	46	At least 2 anterior levels, 1 lateral, and 3 posterior	
Abdominal	47	Helps patient with position changes.	
	48	Covers lower extremities with a sheet during the exam.	
	49	Palpation	**2–3 cm aorta. No masses**
Vascular	50	Palpation of peripheral pulses/capillary refill	**1/4 throughout, cap refill 3 seconds**
Neurologic	51	Motor strength testing with b/l comparison	**5/5 upper and lower extremities b/l**
	52	Reflexes	**2/4 upper and lower extremities b/l**
	53	Cerebellar functioning	**RAM, F/N, H/S, pronator drift intact**
	54	Babinski's sign	**Downgoing**
	55	Romberg	**Negative**
Rectal	56	Advises that rectal exam is recommended.	**Not performed on SP**
Assessment	57	Presents patient with a proposed diagnosis.	**Orthostatic hypotension**
Plan	58	MTHR: d/c HCTZ, labs, imaging, ECG, position change education	
(MOTHRR)	59	Return plan: Devises and explains a follow-up plan with the patient.	
	60	Thanks the patient and asks if there are any questions.	

Humanistic Evaluation   Y/N

Did the candidate present in a self-caring manner (e.g., hair control, clothing, cleanliness, aroma, etc.)?	
Did the candidate make periodic eye contact?	
Was the candidate's language clear and EASY to understand?	
Did the candidate have any substance in his or her mouth during the session?	
Did the candidate exhibit body language that would make you feel the candidate was communicating with you?	
Was the candidate enthusiastic?	
Did the candidate exhibit pride in his or her efforts?	
Did the candidate make any comment regarding your lifestyle (e.g., your work, family, activities, etc.)?	
Did the candidate express any humanistic statement recognizing your concerns?	
Did the candidate explain the medical problem and offer you a possible diagnosis?	
Did the candidate suggest a treatment plan that you could understand?	
Did the candidate inquire whether you might want to consult with family members or others about your visit?	
Did the candidate present as if he or she were a competent interviewer?	
Did the candidate ask you if you had any questions?	
Did the candidate thank you?	

Case 23

Patient Name: Barry Bretten
Clinical Setting: Family Practice Office
CC: A 57 y/o male presents for shortness of breath.

Vital Signs
Blood pressure: 122/68
Respirations: 16 per minute
Temperature: 100.6°F
Pulse: 92 bpm
Weight: 225 lbs
Height: 6'

NOTES:

Subjective

Objective

Assessment

Plan

CC: A 57 y/o male presents for shortness of breath.

History			✓
	1 Introduces self and explains role of provider.		
	2 Properly washes hands before touching the patient (15-sec wash and turns off with towel).		
	3 Opening question: What brings you in today?	I've got this bad cough.	
Chronology/ Onset	4 **When** did this start?	The last week or so.	
	5 Are you **doing anything** when it happens?	No. It's all the time.	
	6 Did you ever have this **before**?	No.	
Description	7 Can you **describe** the cough?	It's wet.	
	8 **Sputum production**?	Yes.	
	9 What **color** is it?	It's thick and rusty looking.	
Intensity	10 How does this affect your **daily activities**?	I can't sleep at night.	
Exacerbation	11 Does anything make it **worse**?	Exerting myself.	
Remission	12 Did you try anything to make it **better**?	Robitussin syrup didn't do a thing.	
	13 How much did you take?	One tablespoon every 4 hours or so.	
Symptoms associated	14 The nurse noted you had **shortness of breath**.	Yes.	
	15 **Chest pain?**	Just when I cough.	
	16 **Fever?**	Yes.	
	17 **Chills?**	A little.	
	18 **Muscle aches?**	Not really.	
	19 **Sore throat?**	A little.	
Social Hx	20 Do you **smoke**?	Yes.	
(FED TACOS)	21 **How much** a day?	About a half pack.	
	22 **How many years?**	About 40 years or so.	
	23 Do you drink **alcohol**?	No.	
	24 Do you drink **caffeine**?	I have couple cups of coffee a day.	
	25 What is your **occupation**?	I'm an author.	
Medical Hx	26 Do you have any medical conditions?	I have high blood pressure.	
Allergies	27 Do you have any allergies?	A little seasonal runny nose.	
Surg Hx	28 Have you had any surgeries?	No.	
Hosp Hx	29 Have you ever been hospitalized?	No.	
Family Hx	30 Medical conditions that run in the family?	High blood pressure and some sugar.	
	31 Do you know what those problems were?	Asthma, I think.	
Medications	32 Are you on any medications?	Hydrochlorothiazide.	
	33 How many pills a day?	One in the morning and one at night.	
	34 How many milligrams?	50 mg.	

Physical Examination ✓

	35	Informs patient that the physical exam is to begin and asks permission.	
	36	Rewashes hand before touching patient if candidate has recontaminated them.	
Gen Assessment	37	Inspection	**Tall, thin, in no apparent distress**
Skin	38	Inspection of skin and nails	**No cyanosis, pallor, or clubbing**
HEENT	39	Inspection	**No pharyngeal erythema/exudate**
Lymphatics	40	Palpation	**No cervical/axillary lymphadenopathy**
Respiratory	41	Inspection: Properly exposes the chest	**No accessory muscle use**
	42	Auscultation performed on bare skin	**Right middle lobe crackles**
	43	Through complete inspiration and expiration	
	44	Symmetrically	
	45	At least 2 anterior levels, 1 lateral, and 3 posterior	
	46	Tactile fremitus	**Increased right middle lobe**
	47	Percussion	**Mild dullness right middle lobe**
Special Testing	48	Egophony, bronchophony, whispered pectoriloquy	**Increased right middle lobe**
Cardiac	49	Auscultation performed on bare skin	**RR without murmurs, rubs, gallops**
	50	Areas: aortic, pulmonic, tricuspid, and mitral	
Assessment	51	Presents patient with a proposed diagnosis.	**Pneumonia**
Plan	52	MTHR: Antibiotic, imaging, labs, smoking cessation, consider admission	
(MOTHRR)	53	Explains and offers OMM.	
	54	Performs OMM appropriately (no HVLA).	
	55	Return plan: Devises and explains a follow-up plan with the patient.	
	56	Thanks the patient and asks if there are any questions.	

Humanistic Evaluation Y/N

Did the candidate present in a self-caring manner (e.g., hair control, clothing, cleanliness, aroma, etc.)?	
Did the candidate make periodic eye contact?	
Was the candidate's language clear and EASY to understand?	
Did the candidate have any substance in his or her mouth during the session?	
Did the candidate exhibit body language that would make you feel the candidate was communicating with you?	
Was the candidate enthusiastic?	
Did the candidate exhibit pride in his or her efforts?	
Did the candidate make any comment regarding your lifestyle (e.g., your work, family, activities, etc.)?	
Did the candidate express any humanistic statement recognizing your concerns?	
Did the candidate explain the medical problem and offer you a possible diagnosis?	
Did the candidate suggest a treatment plan that you could understand?	
Did the candidate inquire whether you might want to consult with family members or others about your visit?	
Did the candidate present as if he or she were a competent interviewer?	
Did the candidate ask you if you had any questions?	
Did the candidate thank you?	

Case 24

Patient Name:	Ruby Todd
Clinical Setting:	Family Practice Office
CC:	A 45 y/o female presents for "swelling of the wrists."

Vital Signs

Blood pressure:	125/78
Respirations:	15 per minute
Temperature:	98.6°F
Pulse:	72 bpm
Weight:	145 lbs
Height:	5'6"

NOTES:

Subjective

Objective

Assessment

Plan

CC: A 45 y/o female presents for "swelling of the wrists."

History			✓
	1	Introduces self and explains role of provider.	
	2	Properly washes hands before touching the patient (15-sec wash and turns off with towel).	
	3	Opening question: What brings you in today?	My wrists and hands are swollen.
Chronology/ Onset	4	**When** did this start?	It started several months ago.
	5	Did you ever have this **before then**?	Just a hint, now and then.
	6	**How often** does it happen?	They're swollen most days now.
	7	Does it come on **suddenly** or **gradually**?	Gradually.
	8	What are you **doing** when it happens?	Nothing really.
Description	9	Could you **describe it**?	I can't get my rings on.
Exacerbation	10	Does anything make it **worse**?	It seems worse in the mornings.
Remission	11	What makes it **better**?	It's better as the day goes on.
Symptoms associated	12	**Stiffness in the mornings?**	Yes.
	13	**Pain in the hands and wrists?**	Yes.
	14	Can you **describe the pain**?	It's an achiness.
	15	Intensity on a scale from 0 to 10?	Seven.
	16	**Other joints** involved?	Sometimes my knees and ankles ache.
	17	**Tired or fatigued?**	All the time.
	18	**Do you feel sad or depressed?**	Not really.
	19	**Weight loss?**	That would be nice.
Social Hx	20	Do you **exercise**?	Yes. I feel better when I do.
(FED TACOS)	21	Do you **smoke or use tobacco**?	Yes.
	22	**How much** a day?	Half a pack a day.
	23	For **how long**?	Twenty-five years.
	24	Do you drink **alcohol**?	No.
	25	What is your **occupation**?	I'm a nurse.
	26	When was the **FDLMP**?	About a week ago.
Medical Hx	27	Do you have any medical conditions?	No.
Allergies	28	Do you have any allergies?	No.
Surgical Hx	29	Have you had any surgeries?	No.
Hosp Hx	30	Have you ever been hospitalized?	No.
Family Hx	31	Medical conditions that run in the family?	My mother has bad arthritis.
Medications	32	Are you on any medications?	Advil.
	33	How much?	I take it once or twice a week.
	34	How many milligrams?	I don't know. Three pills.

Physical Examination ✓

	35	Informs patient that the physical exam is to begin and asks permission.	
	36	Rewashes hands before touching patient if candidate has recontaminated them.	
Eyes	37	Inspection of conjunctiva	**Pink without exudate**
Neck	38	Inspection	**Symmetrical**
Respiratory	39	Auscultation performed on bare skin	**Clear to auscultation**
	40	Through complete inspiration and expiration	
	41	Symmetrically	
	42	At least 2 anterior levels, 1 lateral, and 3 posterior	
Cardiac	43	Auscultation performed on bare skin	**RR without murmurs, rubs, or gallops**
	44	Areas: aortic, pulmonic, tricuspid, and mitral	
MS	45	Wrists and hands: Inspection	**Mild joint erythema, edema. No deformity**
	46	Active range of motion	**Mild AROM limitation**
		Passive range of motion	**Mild pain PROM**
	47	Palpation	**Mild DIP/PIP tenderness and warmth**
	48	Covers patient with a sheet from waist down.	
	49	Knees and ankles: Bilateral inspection	**No edema, erythema, deformity**
	50	Active range of motion	**Full AROM**
	51	Palpation	**Nontender to palpation**
Neurologic	52	Motor strength testing with bilateral comparison	**4/5 fingers, 5/5 otherwise throughout**
	53	Reflexes	**2/4 throughout**
Assessment	54	Presents patient with a proposed diagnosis.	**Rheumatoid arthritis**
Plan	55	MTHR: Pain control, labs (CBC, ESR, RF, ANA), imaging, referral	
(MOTHRR)	56	Explains and offers OMM.	
	57	Performs OMM appropriately (no HVLA).	
	58	Return plan: Devises and explains a follow-up plan with the patient.	
	59	Thanks the patient and asks if there are any questions.	

Humanistic Evaluation Y/N

Did the candidate present in a self-caring manner (e.g., hair control, clothing, cleanliness, aroma, etc.)?	
Did the candidate make periodic eye contact?	
Was the candidate's language clear and EASY to understand?	
Did the candidate have any substance in his or her mouth during the session?	
Did the candidate exhibit body language that would make you feel the candidate was communicating with you?	
Was the candidate enthusiastic?	
Did the candidate exhibit pride in his or her efforts?	
Did the candidate make any comment regarding your lifestyle (e.g., your work, family, activities, etc.)?	
Did the candidate express any humanistic statement recognizing your concerns?	
Did the candidate explain the medical problem and offer you a possible diagnosis?	
Did the candidate suggest a treatment plan that you could understand?	
Did the candidate inquire whether you might want to consult with family members or others about your visit?	
Did the candidate present as if he or she were a competent interviewer?	
Did the candidate ask you if you had any questions?	
Did the candidate thank you?	

Case 25

Patient Name: Elizabeth Barr
Clinical Setting: Family Practice Office
CC: A 20 y/o female presents for "a rash."

Vital Signs
Blood pressure: 110/88
Respirations: 16 per minute
Temperature: 99.2°F
Pulse: 78 bpm
Weight: 118 lbs
Height: 5'3"

NOTES:

Subjective

Objective

Assessment

Plan

CC: A 20 y/o female presents for "a rash."

History				✓
	1	Introduces self and explains role of provider.		
	2	Properly washes hands before touching the patient (15-sec wash and turns off with towel).		
	3	Opening question: What brings you in today?	I have a rash.	
Chronology/ Onset	4	**When** did this start?	Yesterday.	
	5	Did you ever have this **before**?	No.	
Description	6	Could you **describe the rash**?	I have red spots all over.	
	7	Does the rash itch?	Yes.	
Intensity	8	On a scale from 0 to 10?	A 5.	
Exacerbation	9	Does anything make it **worse**?	No.	
Remission	10	What makes it **better**?	Benadryl cream helped a little.	
Symptoms associated	11	**Have you been ill recently?**	Yes, I've had a sore throat.	
	12	**Fever?**	I've felt warm.	
	13	**Nasal discharge?**	No.	
	14	**Ear pain?**	No.	
	15	**Fatigue?**	Yes. I've been very tired.	
	16	**Nausea or vomiting?**	No.	
	17	**Cough?**	No.	
Social Hx	18	Do you **smoke**?	Yes.	
(FED TACOS)	19	**How much** is "a little"?	A half pack a day.	
	20	**How long** have you been smoking?	Two or 3 years.	
	21	Do you drink **alcohol**?	No.	
	22	Do you use any **drugs**?	No.	
	23	What is your **occupation**?	I'm not working. I'm in college.	
	24	**New soaps/detergents/chemicals?**	No.	
	25	**Environmental exposures/outdoors?**	No.	
Medical Hx	26	Do you have any medical conditions?	No.	
Allergies	27	Do you have any allergies?	No.	
Surg Hx	28	Have you had any surgeries?	No.	
Hosp Hx	29	Have you ever been hospitalized?	No.	
Family Hx	30	Medical conditions that run in the family?	No.	
Medications	31	Are you on any medications?	Amoxicillin.	
	32	When were you started on that?	I got it from an Urgent Care 2 days ago.	
	33	For what reason?	For my sore throat.	

Physical Examination ✓

	34	Informs patient that the physical exam is to begin and asks permission.	
	35	Rewashes hands before touching patient if candidate has recontaminated them.	
Skin	36	Inspection/palpation with proper exposure	**Nonblanching, maculopapular rash present on the face and extremities**
Ears	37	External inspection	**No exudate**
	38	Otoscopic examination	**TM's gray b/l**
	39	Inverted otoscope with finger distended	
	40	Proper ear position—Adult: up, back, out	
Nose	41	Inspection with light source	**No discharge**
Throat	42	Inspection with light source and tongue blade	**Erythematous w/white tonsillar exudate**
Lymphatics	43	Palpation of cervical nodes	**Anterior cervical adenopathy b/l**
Respiratory	44	Auscultation performed on bare skin	**Clear to auscultation**
	45	Through complete inspiration and expiration	
	46	Symmetrically	
	47	At least 2 anterior levels, 1 lateral, and 3 posterior	
Cardiac	48	Auscultation performed on bare skin	**RR without murmurs, rubs, or gallops**
	49	Areas: aortic, pulmonic, tricuspid, and mitral	
Abdominal	50	Helps patient with position changes.	
	51	Covers lower extremities with a sheet during the exam.	
	52	Inspection: Properly exposes the abdomen	**Flat**
	53	Auscultation prior to palpation.	**Normoactive bowel sounds**
	54	Palpation	**Nontender. No organomegaly**
Assessment	55	Presents patient with a proposed diagnosis	**Amoxicillin use in likely EBV infection**
Plan	56	MTHR: Stop amoxicillin, throat culture, holistic (contact avoidance), smoking cessation	
(MOTHRR)	57	Return plan: Devises and explains a follow-up plan with the patient.	
	58	Thanks the patient and asks if there are any questions.	

Humanistic Evaluation Y/N

Did the candidate present in a self-caring manner (e.g., hair control, clothing, cleanliness, aroma, etc.)?	
Did the candidate make periodic eye contact?	
Was the candidate's language clear and EASY to understand?	
Did the candidate have any substance in his or her mouth during the session?	
Did the candidate exhibit body language that would make you feel the candidate was communicating with you?	
Was the candidate enthusiastic?	
Did the candidate exhibit pride in his or her efforts?	
Did the candidate make any comment regarding your lifestyle (e.g., your work, family, activities, etc.)?	
Did the candidate express any humanistic statement recognizing your concerns?	
Did the candidate explain the medical problem and offer you a possible diagnosis?	
Did the candidate suggest a treatment plan that you could understand?	
Did the candidate inquire whether you might want to consult with family members or others about your visit?	
Did the candidate present as if he or she were a competent interviewer?	
Did the candidate ask you if you had any questions?	
Did the candidate thank you?	

Case 26

Patient Name: Kali Moto
Clinical Setting: Family Practice Office
CC: A 14 y/o female presents for "a hump on her back." Mother is present.

Vital Signs:
Blood pressure: 98/70
Respirations: 12 per minute
Temperature: 98°F
Pulse: 82 bpm
Weight: 115 lbs
Height: 4' 10"

NOTES:

Subjective

Objective

Assessment

Plan

CC: A 14 y/o female presents for "a hump on her back."

		History		✓
	1	Introduces self and explains role of provider.		
	2	Properly washes hands before touching the patient (15-sec wash and turns off with towel).		
	3	Opening question: What brings you in today?	My mom said I have a hump on my back.	
Onset	4	**When** was this?	She noticed it last week.	
Chronology	5	Did you ever have this **before**?	No.	
Exacerbation	6	Does anything make it **worse**?	Not really.	
Remission	7	What makes it **better**?	I don't know.	
Symptoms associated	8	**Back pain**?	A little.	
	9	Where?	Mostly between my shoulder blades.	
	10	Intensity from 1 to 10?	A 3.	
	11	**Muscle weakness?**	No.	
	12	**Numbness or tingling?**	No.	
	13	**Bowel or bladder problems?**	No.	
	14	**Headache?**	No.	
	15	**Neck pain?**	No.	
	16	**Shortness of breath, difficulty breathing?**	No.	
	17	**Recent growth?**	I think a few inches.	
Social Hx	18	Do you **exercise**?	I play soccer.	
(FED TACOS)	19	Do you **smoke**?	No.	
	20	Do you drink **alcohol**?	No.	
	21	Use any **drugs**?	No.	
	22	Do you **work**?	No. I just go to school.	
	23	When was the **FDLMP**?	About 3 weeks ago.	
Medical Hx	24	Do you have any medical conditions?	No.	
	25	Lower limb fracture, joint infection, arthritis?	No	
Allergies	26	Do you have any allergies?	No.	
Surg Hx	27	Have you had any surgeries?	No.	
Hosp Hx	28	Have you ever been hospitalized?	No.	
Family Hx	29	Conditions/joint problems in the family?	None that I know of.	
Medications	30	Are you on any medications?	No.	

Physical Examination ✓

	31	Informs patient that the physical exam is to begin and asks permission.	
	32	Rewashes hands before touching patient if candidate has recontaminated them.	
Cardiac	33	Auscultation performed on bare skin	**Regular rhythm w/o murmur, rub, gallop**
	34	Areas: aortic, pulmonic, tricuspid, and mitral	
Respiratory	35	Auscultation performed on bare skin	**Clear to auscultation**
	36	Through complete inspiration and expiration	
	37	Symmetrically	
	38	At least 2 anterior levels, 1 lateral, and 3 posterior	
Musculoskeletal	39	Assists patient to standing position.	
	40	Inspection: Gown open in back, with undergarments that expose the iliac crests and posterior and anterior superior iliac spines	**R shoulder slightly higher than L. No cafe au lait, axillary freckling, dimpling, or hair patches**
	41	Lateral view	**Decreased thoracic kyphosis**
	42	Forward bend test: Feet together, knees straight ahead, and arms hanging free	**T5–11 RrSr**
	43	Feet	**Arches are intact.**
	44	AROM followed by PROM	**Decreased thoracic sidebend L, rotate L**
	45	Measurement of leg lengths	**Leg lengths are equal.**
Neurologic	46	Motor strength testing—b/l comparison	**Intact 5/5 upper and lower extremities**
	47	Sensory: Sharp dull, light touch	**Intact upper and lower extremities b/l**
	48	Reflexes	**2/4 upper and lower extremities b/l**
Assessment	49	Presents patient with a proposed diagnosis.	**Scoliosis. Somatic dysfunction**
Plan	50	MTHR: Pain control, holistic (exercises), imaging, referral	
(MOTHRR)	51	Explains and offers OMM.	
	52	Performs OMM appropriately (no HVLA).	
	53	Return plan: Devises and explains a follow-up plan with the patient.	
	54	Thanks the patient and mother. Asks if there are any questions.	

Humanistic Evaluation Y/N

Did the candidate present in a self-caring manner (e.g., hair control, clothing, cleanliness, aroma, etc.)?	
Did the candidate make periodic eye contact?	
Was the candidate's language clear and EASY to understand?	
Did the candidate have any substance in his or her mouth during the session?	
Did the candidate exhibit body language that would make you feel the candidate was communicating with you?	
Was the candidate enthusiastic?	
Did the candidate exhibit pride in his or her efforts?	
Did the candidate make any comment regarding your lifestyle (e.g., your work, family, activities, etc.)?	
Did the candidate express any humanistic statement recognizing your concerns?	
Did the candidate explain the medical problem and offer you a possible diagnosis?	
Did the candidate suggest a treatment plan that you could understand?	
Did the candidate inquire whether you might want to consult with family members or others about your visit?	
Did the candidate present as if he or she were a competent interviewer?	
Did the candidate ask you if you had any questions?	
Did the candidate thank you?	

Case 27

Patient Name:	Stephanie Dubb
Clinical Setting:	Family Practice Office
CC:	A 36 y/o female presents for "a cold."

Vital Signs

Blood pressure:	118/128
Respirations:	16 per minute
Temperature:	100.2°F
Pulse:	88 bpm
Weight:	128 lbs
Height:	5'5"

NOTES:

Subjective

Objective

Assessment

Plan

CC: A 36 y/o female presents for "a cold."

History			✓
	1 Introduces self and explains role of provider.		
	2 Properly washes hands before touching the patient (15-sec wash and turns off with towel).		
	3 Opening question: What brings you in today?	I've got a cold.	
Chronology/ Onset	4 **When** did this start?	Three days ago.	
	5 How has it **changed**?	It seems to be getting worse.	
	6 Did you ever have this **before**?	Yes.	
	7 **How often** does it happen?	About once a year.	
	8 How was it **treated**?	I think they gave me antibiotics.	
Description	9 Could you **describe the cold**?	My nose is all stuffed up and I'm coughing.	
Exacerbation	10 Does anything make it **worse**?	Lying flat.	
Remission	11 What makes it **better**?	A hot shower helps a little.	
Symptoms associated	12 **Sinus congestion/pressure?**	Yes.	
	13 **Do you have a headache?**	Yes.	
	14 Location?	*Points to frontal sinuses*	
	15 **Nasal discharge?**	Yes.	
	16 What **color** is it?	It was clear, now it's green and smells bad.	
	17 **Fever?**	I haven't taken my temperature.	
	18 **Ear pain?**	It feels like they are blocked up.	
	19 **Sore throat?**	Not really.	
	20 **Postnasal drainage?**	Yes.	
	21 **Ear pain?**	No, they just feel full.	
	22 **Cough?**	No.	
Social Hx	23 Do you **smoke**?	Yes.	
(FED TACOS)	24 **How much** a day?	About a pack a day.	
	25 **How many years?**	About 15.	
	26 Do you drink **alcohol**?	No.	
	27 Do you use any **drugs**?	No.	
	28 What is your **occupation**?	I'm a teacher.	
Medical Hx	29 Do you have any medical conditions?	No.	
Allergies	30 Do you have any **allergies**?	No.	
Surg Hx	31 Have you had any surgeries?	No.	
Hosp Hx	32 Have you ever been hospitalized?	No.	
Family Hx	33 Medical conditions that run in the family?	Nothing in particular.	
	34 Anyone you know with the same symptoms?	Some of the kids at school have been sick.	
Menstrual Hx	35 When was the **FDLMP**?	A couple of weeks ago.	
Medications	36 Are you on any medications?	No.	

Physical Examination ✓

	37	Informs patient that the physical exam is to begin and asks permission.		
	38	Rewashes hand before touching patient if candidate has recontaminated them.		
Sinuses	39	Palpation/percussion	**Tenderness of the frontal sinuses**	
Eyes	40	Inspection	**No periorbital edema noted**	
Ears	41	Inspection: External	**No exudate**	
	42	Depresses tragus/retracts pinna for pain	**No pain**	
	43	Otoscopic examination	**TM's gray b/l**	
	44	Inverted otoscope with finger distended		
	45	Proper position: Up, back, out		
Nose	46	Inspection	**Purulent nasal discharge**	
Throat	47	Inspection with light source and tongue blade	**Purulent postnasal drip present**	
Lymphatics	48	Palpation: Cervical	**No lymphadenopathy**	
Respiratory	49	Auscultation performed on bare skin	**Clear to auscultation**	
	50	Through complete inspiration and expiration		
	51	Symmetrically		
	52	At least 2 anterior levels, 1 lateral, and 3 posterior		
Cardiac	53	Auscultation performed on bare skin	**RR without murmurs, rubs, or gallops**	
	54	Areas: aortic, pulmonic, tricuspid, and mitral		
Assessment	55	Presents patient with a proposed diagnosis.	**Sinusitis**	
Plan	56	MTHR: Antibiotics, increase fluids, rest, remain off work, smoking cessation		
(MOTHRR)	57	Return plan: Devises and explains a follow-up plan with the patient.		
	58	Thanks the patient and asks if there are any questions.		

Humanistic Evaluation Y/N

Did the candidate present in a self-caring manner (e.g., hair control, clothing, cleanliness, aroma, etc.)?	
Did the candidate make periodic eye contact?	
Was the candidate's language clear and EASY to understand?	
Did the candidate have any substance in his or her mouth during the session?	
Did the candidate exhibit body language that would make you feel the candidate was communicating with you?	
Was the candidate enthusiastic?	
Did the candidate exhibit pride in his or her efforts?	
Did the candidate make any comment regarding your lifestyle (e.g., your work, family, activities, etc.)?	
Did the candidate express any humanistic statement recognizing your concerns?	
Did the candidate explain the medical problem and offer you a possible diagnosis?	
Did the candidate suggest a treatment plan that you could understand?	
Did the candidate inquire whether you might want to consult with family members or others about your visit?	
Did the candidate present as if he or she were a competent interviewer?	
Did the candidate ask you if you had any questions?	
Did the candidate thank you?	

Case 28

Patient Name:	Carrie Mei
Clinical Setting:	Primary Care Outpatient Office Visit
CC:	A 56 y/o female presents c/o lower leg pain.

Vital Signs

Blood pressure:	112/58
Respirations:	12 per minute
Temperature:	98.8°F
Pulse:	72 bpm
Weight:	167 lbs
Height:	5'4"

NOTES:

Subjective

Objective

Assessment

Plan

CC: A 56 y/o female presents c/o lower leg pain.

History			✓
	1 Introduces self and explains role of provider.		
	2 Properly washes hands before touching the patient (15-sec wash and turns off with towel).		
	3 Opening question: What brings you in today?	I hurt my leg.	
Onset	4 **When** did it happen?	Yesterday.	
	5 **How/what** were you **doing** at the time?	I was standing on my toes, lifting a TV.	
Chronology	6 Has this ever happened **before**?	Yes.	
	7 **When?**	About 20 years ago.	
	8 **Prior diagnosis?**	I had a partially torn tendon.	
	9 **How was it treated?**	I had 4 weeks of physical therapy.	
Description/	10 **Where** is the pain?	Behind my right ankle. (*Touches Achilles*)	
Duration	11 **Describe** the pain.	I heard a loud pop and had a sudden pain.	
Intensity	12 How severe is it, on a scale from **1 to 10**?	At least an 8.	
Exacerbation	13 What makes it **worse**?	Trying to walk on it.	
Remission	14 What makes it **better**?	Ibuprofen helps.	
	15 **How much** did you take?	Three tablets.	
	16 How **often** are you taking them?	Every 3 hours.	
Symptoms associated	17 **Bruising?**	Yes, a lot.	
	18 **Swelling?**	It was swollen last night.	
	19 **Weakness?**	Yes. I can't stand up on my right toes.	
Social Hx	20 Do you **smoke** or **use tobacco**?	No.	
(FED TACOS)	21 Do you drink **alcohol**?	Yes.	
	22 **How much** a day?	One glass of wine a day with dinner.	
	23 What is your **occupation**?	I volunteer at the Veterans Hospital.	
Medical Hx	24 Do you have any medical conditions?	I have high cholesterol.	
Allergies	25 Do you have any allergies?	No.	
Surgical Hx	26 Have you had any surgeries?	No.	
Hosp Hx	27 Have you ever been hospitalized?	No.	
Family Hx	28 Medical conditions that run in the family?	We all have high cholesterol.	
Medications	29 Are you on any medications?	Lovastatin.	
	30 How much?	80 mg once a day.	

Physical Examination ✓

	31	Informs patient that the physical exam is to begin and asks permission.	
	32	Rewashes hand before touching patient if candidate has recontaminated them.	
MS	33	Inspection	**Right posterior ankle ecchymosis**
	34	Covers patient with a sheet from waist down.	**Right foot hangs down.**
	35	Raises sheet to expose bilateral lower extremities.	
	36	Active range of motion right ankle	**Cannot plantarflex**
	37	Passive range of motion	**Full range of motion**
	38	Palpation	**Tenderness right posterior Achilles**
Vascular	39	Palpation—peripheral pulses	**Dorsalis pedis/posterior tib 2/4 b/l**
Neurologic	40	Strength testing—at ankles bilaterally	**0/4 Right plantarflexion**
Position change	41	Helps patient with position change to standing.	
	42	Assesses gait.	**Patient walks with flat foot on right.**
Assessment	43	Presents patient with a proposed diagnosis.	**Achilles injury, sprain or rupture**
Plan	44	MTHR: Pain control (reduce ibuprofen), testing, holistic (RICE), referral	
(MOTHRR)	45	Explains and offers OMM.	
	46	Performs OMM appropriately (no HVLA).	
	47	Return plan: Devises and explains a follow-up plan with the patient.	
	48	Thanks the patient and asks if there are any questions.	

Humanistic Evaluation Y/N

Did the candidate present in a self-caring manner (e.g., hair control, clothing, cleanliness, aroma, etc.)?	
Did the candidate make periodic eye contact?	
Was the candidate's language clear and EASY to understand?	
Did the candidate have any substance in his or her mouth during the session?	
Did the candidate exhibit body language that would make you feel the candidate was communicating with you?	
Was the candidate enthusiastic?	
Did the candidate exhibit pride in his or her efforts?	
Did the candidate make any comment regarding your lifestyle (e.g., your work, family, activities, etc.)?	
Did the candidate express any humanistic statement recognizing your concerns?	
Did the candidate explain the medical problem and offer you a possible diagnosis?	
Did the candidate suggest a treatment plan that you could understand?	
Did the candidate inquire whether you might want to consult with family members or others about your visit?	
Did the candidate present as if he or she were a competent interviewer?	
Did the candidate ask you if you had any questions?	
Did the candidate thank you?	

Patient Name: Melissa Mencies
Clinical Setting: Family Practice Outpatient Office Visit
CC: A 22 y/o female complaining of no menses for 3 months.

Vital Signs
Blood pressure: 110/60
Respirations: 12 per minute
Temperature: 98.9°F
Pulse: 68 bpm
Weight: 105 lbs
Height: 5'4"

NOTES:

Subjective

Objective

Assessment

Plan

CC: A 22 y/o female complaining of no menses for 3 months.

History				✓
	1	Introduces self and explains role of provider.		
	2	Properly washes hands before touching the patient (15-sec wash and turns off with towel).		
	3	Opening question: What brings you in today?	I haven't had my period.	
Chronology/ Onset	4	When was the **first day of your last menstrual period**?	About 4 months ago.	
	5	Have you ever **missed a period before**?	No.	
	6	Have your periods **changed** at all before this?	No.	
Obstetric Hx	7	**Age at first period**?	Thirteen.	
	8	Were your periods **regular before this**?	Yes.	
	9	How many **days apart** are they normally?	About 25.	
	10	How **long** do they **last**?	About 3 days.	
	11	Describe the **flow** as heavy, medium, or light.	Light each day.	
Sexual Hx	12	Are you **sexually active**?	Yes.	
	13	Do you use **protection**?	Yes.	
	14	What **form of protection** do you use?	We use the rhythmic cycle.	
	15	Have you ever been **pregnant**?	No.	
Symptoms associated	16	**Discharge from the breasts?**	No.	
	17	**Breast tenderness or enlargement?**	They are a little sore.	
	18	**Nausea or vomiting?**	I am nauseated a lot lately.	
	19	**Fatigue, cold intolerance, weight gain?**	No.	
	20	**Abdominal pain?**	No.	
	21	**Visual changes?**	No.	
Social Hx	22	How is your **diet**?	I'm vegetarian.	
	23	How much do you **exercise**?	I run 10 miles a day.	
	24	Do you **smoke**?	No.	
	25	Do you **drink**?	No.	
	26	Do you use any **drugs**?	No.	
	27	What is your **occupation**?	I'm a yoga instructor.	
Medical Hx	28	Do you have any medical conditions?	No.	
Allergies	29	Do you have any allergies?	No.	
Surg Hx	30	Have you had any surgeries?	No.	
Hosp Hx	31	Have you ever been hospitalized?	No.	
Family Hx	32	Medical conditions that run in the family?	My father has prostate cancer.	
Medications	33	Are you on any medications?	No.	

Physical Examination ✓

	34	Informs patient that the physical exam is to begin and asks permission.	
	35	Rewashes hands before touching patient if candidate has recontaminated them.	
General	36	General assessment	**Alert, timid, thin**
Skin	37	Assesses hair texture/pattern and skin texture.	**Normal**
HEENT	38	Assesses for facial hair.	**None**
Neck	39	Palpates the thyroid.	**No thyromegaly or nodules**
Respiratory	40	Auscultation performed on bare skin	**Clear to auscultation**
	41	Through complete inspiration and expiration	
	42	Symmetrically	
	43	At least 2 anterior levels, 1 lateral, and 3 posterior	
Cardiac	44	Auscultation performed on bare skin	**RR without murmurs, rubs, gallops**
	45	Areas: aortic, pulmonic, tricuspid, and mitral	
Abdomen	46	Inspection	**Slight infraumbilical protuberance**
	47	Auscultation	**Normoactive bowel sounds**
	48	Percussion	**Dullness below the umbilicus**
	49	Palpation	**Uterine fundus to 18 cm**
Genital	50	Advises SP that pelvic exam is recommended.	**Not performed on SP**
Breast	51	Advises SP that breast exam is recommended.	**Not performed on SP**
Assessment	52	Presents patient with a proposed diagnosis.	**Pregnancy**
Plan	53	MTHR: Lab work including pregnancy test, emotional impact evaluation, referral	
(MOTHRR)	54	Return plan: Devises and explains a follow-up plan with the patient.	
	55	Thanks the patient and asks if there are any questions.	

Humanistic Evaluation Y/N

	Y/N
Did the candidate present in a self-caring manner (e.g., hair control, clothing, cleanliness, aroma, etc.)?	
Did the candidate make periodic eye contact?	
Was the candidate's language clear and EASY to understand?	
Did the candidate have any substance in his or her mouth during the session?	
Did the candidate exhibit body language that would make you feel the candidate was communicating with you?	
Was the candidate enthusiastic?	
Did the candidate exhibit pride in his or her efforts?	
Did the candidate make any comment regarding your lifestyle (e.g., your work, family, activities, etc.)?	
Did the candidate express any humanistic statement recognizing your concerns?	
Did the candidate explain the medical problem and offer you a possible diagnosis?	
Did the candidate suggest a treatment plan that you could understand?	
Did the candidate inquire whether you might want to consult with family members or others about your visit?	
Did the candidate present as if he or she were a competent interviewer?	
Did the candidate ask you if you had any questions?	
Did the candidate thank you?	

Case 30

Patient Name: Terry O'Pen
Clinical Setting: Emergency Room
CC: A 22 y/o male college student presents with chest pain.

Vital Signs
Blood pressure: 180/100
Respirations: 24 per minute
Temperature: 98.8°F
Pulse: 110 bpm
Weight: 190 lbs
Height: 6'6"

NOTES:

Subjective

Objective

Assessment

Plan

CC: A 22 y/o male college student presents with chest pain.

History			✓
	1	Introduces self and explains role of provider.	
	2	Properly washes hands before touching the patient (15-sec wash and turns off with towel).	
	3	Opening question: What brings you in today?	I have chest pain.	
Chronology/ Onset	4	When did it **start**?	About an hour ago.	
	5	What were you **doing**?	Playing basketball.	
	6	Did you ever have this **before**?	No.	
Description/ Duration	7	**Describe** the pain.	It's a ripping, a tearing.	
	8	**Where** is the pain?	In the center of my chest.	
	9	Does it **radiate** anywhere?	Between my shoulder blades.	
	10	Was the onset **sudden** or **gradual**?	It happened all of a sudden.	
	11	Is it **continuous** or does it **come and go**?	Continuous.	
Intensity	12	How severe is it, on a scale from **1 to 10**?	An 8.	
Exacerbation	13	What makes it **worse**?	Nothing.	
Remission	14	What makes it **better**?	Nothing.	
Symptoms associated	15	**Lightheadedness?**	Yes.	
	16	**Nausea or vomiting?**	No.	
	17	**Shortness of breath/cough?**	Yes.	
	18	**Abdominal pain?**	No.	
	19	**Arms or legs hurt?**	No.	
	20	**Slurred speech, facial droop?**	No.	
	21	**Weakness** or **numbness/tingling?**	My right arm feels heavy.	
Social Hx	22	Do you **smoke**?	No.	
	23	Do you drink **alcohol**?	No.	
	24	Do you use any **drugs**?	Once in a while.	
	25	What do you use?	A little crack on weekends.	
	26	When was the **last time** you **used**?	A couple of days ago.	
Medical Hx	27	Do you have any medical conditions?	I have Marfan's syndrome.	
Allergies	28	Do you have any allergies?	No.	
Surg Hx	29	Have you had any surgeries?	No.	
Hosp Hx	30	Have you ever been hospitalized?	No.	
Family Hx	31	Medical conditions that run in the family?	Arthritis seems to run in the family.	
Medications	32	What **medications** are you on?	None.	

Physical Examination ✓

	33	Informs patient that the physical exam is to begin and asks permission.	
	34	Rewashes hands before touching patient if candidate has recontaminated them.	
Vitals	35	Compares BP bilateral upper extremities.	**Right arm 190/110, Left arm 150/100**
	36	Appropriate size cuff	
	37	Applied correctly placing cuff on bare arm	
	38	Pulse—rate and rhythm	**Regular at 110 bpm**
	39	Respirations—rate	**24 bpm**
General	40	Assesses for **distress**.	**Facial grimaces of distress**
Neck	41	Assesses for **JVD**.	**No JVD**
Cardiac	42	Inspection: Properly exposes the chest	**No heave noted**
	43	Auscultation performed on bare skin	**Grade 2/6 aortic regurgitant murmur**
	44	Areas: aortic, pulmonic, tricuspid, and mitral	
	45	Palpation for PMI	**5th ICS MCL**
Respiratory	46	Auscultation performed on bare skin	**Clear to auscultation**
	47	Through complete inspiration and expiration	
	48	Symmetrically	
	49	At least 2 anterior levels, 1 lateral, and 3 posterior	
	50	Palpation for reproducibility of pain	**Not reproducible**
Extremities	51	Inspection for pallor	**None**
	52	Palpation for peripheral pulses	**3/4 Right arm, 2/4 Left arm**
Neurologic	53	Cranial nerve examination	**CN II–XII intact**
	54	Strength and comparing bilateral extremities	**Equal throughout at 5/5**
Assessment	55	Presents patient with a proposed diagnosis.	**Aortic dissection**
Plan	56	MTHR: Blood pressure control, imaging, EKG, surgical consult	
(MOTHRR)	57	Advises admission and emergent evaluation.	
	58	Thanks the patient and asks if there are any questions.	

Humanistic Evaluation Y/N

Did the candidate present in a self-caring manner (e.g., hair control, clothing, cleanliness, aroma, etc.)?	
Did the candidate make periodic eye contact?	
Was the candidate's language clear and EASY to understand?	
Did the candidate have any substance in his or her mouth during the session?	
Did the candidate exhibit body language that would make you feel the candidate was communicating with you?	
Was the candidate enthusiastic?	
Did the candidate exhibit pride in his or her efforts?	
Did the candidate make any comment regarding your lifestyle (e.g., your work, family, activities, etc.)?	
Did the candidate express any humanistic statement recognizing your concerns?	
Did the candidate explain the medical problem and offer you a possible diagnosis?	
Did the candidate suggest a treatment plan that you could understand?	
Did the candidate inquire whether you might want to consult with family members or others about your visit?	
Did the candidate present as if he or she were a competent interviewer?	
Did the candidate ask you if you had any questions?	
Did the candidate thank you?	

Case 31

Patient Name: Barry Pean
Clinical Setting: Family Practice Outpatient Office Visit
CC: An 82 y/o male presents with a "private problem."

Vital Signs
Blood pressure: 158/72
Respirations: 12 per minute
Temperature: 97.2°F
Pulse: 60 bpm
Weight: 145 lbs
Height: 5'7"

NOTES:

Subjective

Objective

Assessment

Plan

CC: An 82 y/o male presents with a "private problem."

History		✓
	1 Introduces self and explains role of provider.	
	2 Properly washes hands before touching the patient (15-sec wash and turns off with towel).	
	3 Opening question: What brings you in today?	I ain't peein' right.
Chronology/ Onset	4 **When** did it first **start**?	A couple a days ago.
	5 Did this ever happen **before**?	No.
	6 Has it **changed** in any way?	Well, it's harder to get it out.
Description	7 Define **"not peeing right"**?	It's hurtin' when it comes out.
	8 **Describe** the pain.	It's burnin'.
Intensity	9 How severe is it, on a scale from **1 to 10**?	Oh, a 3 or so.
Exacerbation	10 What makes it **worse**?	Nothin' I know of.
Remission	11 What makes it **better**?	Nothin' I know of.
Symptoms associated	12 Is it hard to **get it started**?	Yea, I gotta stand there for a while.
	13 Is it hard to **get it stopped**?	Yea, it dribbles a bit at the end.
	14 **Penile discharge?**	No.
	15 **Blood?**	Well, it looks kinda pink, I'd say.
	16 **Frequency?**	I seem to go a lot.
	17 **Nocturia?**	I get up four or five times a night.
	18 **Change in stream?**	I can't write my name in the snow.
	19 **Fever or chills?**	No. I don't think so.
	20 **Abdominal pain or back pain?**	My bladder feels full, that's all.
Social Hx	21 Do you **smoke**?	No.
	22 Do you drink **alcohol**?	I have a shot now and then.
	23 How often?	Just one blackberry brandy at bedtime.
	24 Do you drink **caffeine**?	I like my coffee.
	25 How much do you drink a day?	Five or six cups.
	26 What is your **occupation**?	I am retired from the railroad 30 years now.
	27 Are you **sexually active**?	Don't I wish.
Medical Hx	28 Do you have any medical conditions?	Just the blood pressure.
Allergies	29 Do you have any allergies?	No.
Surg Hx	30 Have you had any surgeries?	Broke an arm once.
Hosp Hx	31 Have you ever been hospitalized?	No.
Family Hx	32 Medical conditions that run in the family?	Most of 'em die of old age.
Medications	33 Are you on any medications?	Atenolol, when I want to take it.
	34 How often do you take it?	Oh, a couple days a week, I suppose.
	35 How many milligrams is it?	25 mg.
	36 How often are you supposed to take it?	Twice a day.

Physical Examination ✓

	37	Informs patient that the physical exam is to begin and asks permission.	
	38	Rewashes hands before touching patient if candidate has recontaminated them.	
Vitals	39	Repeats BP with correct technique.	**152/70 right arm**
	40	Appropriate size cuff	
	41	Applied correctly placing cuff on bare arm	
General	42	Assesses for **distress**.	**No apparent distress**
Cardiac	43	Auscultation performed on bare skin	**Regular rhythm w/o murmur, rub, gallop**
	44	Areas: aortic, pulmonic, tricuspid, and mitral	
Respiratory	45	Auscultation performed on bare skin	**Clear to auscultation**
	46	Through complete inspiration and expiration	
	47	Symmetrically	
	48	At least 2 anterior levels, 1 lateral, and 3 posterior	
Abdomen	49	Inspection	**Flat without masses**
	50	Auscultation prior to palpation	**Normoactive bowel sounds**
	51	Palpation	**No masses or tenderness**
	52	Percussion	**No bladder distension**
	53	CVA tenderness	**Negative**
Genital	54	Advises SP that genital would be performed.	**Genital exam NOT performed on SP.**
Rectal	55	Advises SP that rectal would be performed.	**Rectal exam NOT performed on SP.**
Assessment	56	Presents patient with a proposed diagnosis.	**Urinary tract infection, BPH**
Plan	57	MTHR: Labs with urinalysis, antibiotic, rectal exam, possible BPH medication	
(MOTHRR)	58	Return plan: Devises and explains a follow-up plan with the patient.	
	59	Thanks the patient and asks if there are any questions.	

Humanistic Evaluation Y/N

Did the candidate present in a self-caring manner (e.g., hair control, clothing, cleanliness, aroma, etc.)?	
Did the candidate make periodic eye contact?	
Was the candidate's language clear and EASY to understand?	
Did the candidate have any substance in his or her mouth during the session?	
Did the candidate exhibit body language that would make you feel the candidate was communicating with you?	
Was the candidate enthusiastic?	
Did the candidate exhibit pride in his or her efforts?	
Did the candidate make any comment regarding your lifestyle (e.g., your work, family, activities, etc.)?	
Did the candidate express any humanistic statement recognizing your concerns?	
Did the candidate explain the medical problem and offer you a possible diagnosis?	
Did the candidate suggest a treatment plan that you could understand?	
Did the candidate inquire whether you might want to consult with family members or others about your visit?	
Did the candidate present as if he or she were a competent interviewer?	
Did the candidate ask you if you had any questions?	
Did the candidate thank you?	

Case 32

Patient Name: Harley Brethin
Clinical Setting: Family Practice Outpatient Office Visit
CC: A 67 y/o Caucasian male presents with a cough.

Vital Signs
Blood pressure: 110/50
Respirations: 24 per minute
Temperature: 101°F
Pulse: 112 bpm
Weight: 232 lbs
Height: 6'

NOTES:

Subjective

Objective

Assessment

Plan

CC: A 67 y/o Caucasian male presents with a cough.

History			✓
	1	Introduces self and explains role of provider.	
	2	Properly washes hands before touching the patient (15-sec wash and turns off with towel).	
	3	Opening question: What brings you in today?	I have a cough.	
Chronology/ Onset	4	When did it **start**?	It crept up on me about a month ago.	
	5	Has it **changed** since it started?	It keeps me up at night now.	
	6	Did you ever have this **before**?	No.	
Description/ Duration	7	**Describe** the cough.	It's wet.	
	8	Are you **bringing up** anything?	Yes.	
	9	What **color** is it?	White or yellow.	
Intensity	10	How has it affected your **ADLs**?	I hang around the house mostly.	
Exacerbation	11	Does anything make it **worse**?	It seems worse in the evening.	
Remission	12	Does anything make it **better**?	Cough medicine hasn't worked.	
	13	What was the **name** of it?	It was some over-the-counter stuff.	
	14	How **much** do you take?	One tablespoon every couple of hours.	
Symptoms associated	15	**Runny nose?**	No.	
	16	**Sore throat?**	Maybe a little.	
	17	**Fever** or **chills?**	I feel a little warm.	
	18	**Chest pain?**	My ribs hurt when I cough.	
	19	**Wheezing?**	I don't think so.	
	20	**Shortness of breath/dyspnea on exertion?**	I get winded just going to the kitchen.	
	21	**Shortness of breath lying flat?**	Yes, I sleep in the recliner.	
	22	**Waking up suddenly SOB (PND)?**	No.	
Social Hx	23	What does your **diet** look like?	I try to avoid the salt.	
(FED TACOS)	24	Do you **exercise**?	No. I get too short of breath to exercise.	
	25	Do you **smoke**?	I used to.	
	26	**When** did you **quit**?	Two weeks ago.	
	27	**How much** did you smoke a day?	One pack a day.	
	28	**How long** had you been smoking?	For 50 years.	
	29	Do you drink **alcohol**?	No.	
	30	What is your **occupation**?	I'm a retired car salesman.	
Medical Hx	31	Do you have any medical conditions?	I have high blood pressure.	
Allergies	32	Do you have any allergies?	No.	
Surg Hx	33	Have you had any surgeries?	No.	
Hosp Hx	34	Have you ever been hospitalized?	I had pneumonia once.	
	35	**When** was that?	About 5 years ago.	
Family Hx	36	Does anything run in the family?	Heart problems.	
Medications	37	What **medications** are you on?	They started lisinopril a month ago.	
	38	How many **milligrams**?	I believe it's 25 twice a day.	

Physical Examination ✓

	39	Informs patient that the physical exam is to begin and asks permission.	
	40	Rewashes hands before touching patient if candidate has recontaminated them.	
Vitals	41	Correctly repeats pulse.	**Regular at 112 bpm**
General	42	Inspection	**Mild accessory muscle use**
Skin	43	Inspection	**No cyanosis**
HEENT	44	Inspection of throat	**No pharyngeal erythema, exudate**
Neck	45	Inspection	**3 cm JVD without thyromegaly**
	46	Auscultation	**No carotid bruit**
	47	Palpation	**No thyromegaly**
Cardiac	48	Inspection: Properly exposes the chest	**No heave or visible PMI**
	49	Auscultation performed on bare skin	**Reg rhythm, S3 without murmur**
	50	Areas: aortic, pulmonic, tricuspid, and mitral	
	51	Palpation for PMI	**Cannot be detected**
Respiratory	52	Inspection	**1:1.5 AP/Lateral diameter**
	53	Auscultation performed on bare skin	**Diminished basilar breath sounds**
	54	Through complete inspiration and expiration	**Crackles bilateral lower lobes**
	55	Symmetrically	
	56	At least 2 anterior levels, 1 lateral, and 3 posterior	
	57	Palpation	**Increased tactile fremitus in bases**
	58	Percussion	**Dullness to percussion in the bases**
Extremities	59	Inspection	**2+ peripheral edema**
Assessment	60	Presents patient with a proposed diagnosis.	**Heart failure**
Plan	61	MTHR: Refers patient to ER for possible admission.	
(MOTHRR)	62	Advises admission and cardiac evaluation.	
	63	Thanks the patient and asks if there are any questions.	

Humanistic Evaluation Y/N

Did the candidate present in a self-caring manner (e.g., hair control, clothing, cleanliness, aroma, etc.)?	
Did the candidate make periodic eye contact?	
Was the candidate's language clear and EASY to understand?	
Did the candidate have any substance in his or her mouth during the session?	
Did the candidate exhibit body language that would make you feel the candidate was communicating with you?	
Was the candidate enthusiastic?	
Did the candidate exhibit pride in his or her efforts?	
Did the candidate make any comment regarding your lifestyle (e.g., your work, family, activities, etc.)?	
Did the candidate express any humanistic statement recognizing your concerns?	
Did the candidate explain the medical problem and offer you a possible diagnosis?	
Did the candidate suggest a treatment plan that you could understand?	
Did the candidate inquire whether you might want to consult with family members or others about your visit?	
Did the candidate present as if he or she were a competent interviewer?	
Did the candidate ask you if you had any questions?	
Did the candidate thank you?	

Patient Name: Gale Stoner
Clinical Setting: Family Practice Outpatient Office Visit
CC: A 43 y/o Caucasian female presents for abdominal pain.

Vital Signs
Blood pressure: 138/85
Respirations: 16 per minute
Temperature: 100.8°F
Pulse: 78 bpm
Weight: 189 lbs
Height: 5' 4"

NOTES:

Subjective

Objective

Assessment

Plan

CC: A 43 y/o Caucasian female presents for abdominal pain.

History			✓
	1 Introduces self and explains role of provider.		
	2 Properly washes hands before touching the patient (15-sec wash and turns off with towel).		
	3 Opening question: What brings you in today?	My stomach hurts.	
Chronology/ Onset	4 When did it **start**?	Last night.	
	5 What were you **doing**?	Just sitting at home.	
	6 Did you ever have this **before**?	Yes.	
	7 When?	On and off for about 6 months.	
Description	8 Was the onset **sudden** or **gradual**?	Gradual.	
Duration	9 Is it **continuous** or does it **come and go**?	Continuous since last night.	
	10 **Describe** the pain.	Like a cramping.	
	11 **Where** is the pain?	*Points to right upper quadrant*	
	12 Does it **radiate** anywhere?	Kind of goes into my back.	
	13 **Where** in the back?	*Points to right scapula*	
Intensity	14 How severe is it, on a scale from **1 to 10**?	An 8.	
Exacerbation	15 What makes it **worse**?	Eating.	
Remission	16 What makes it **better**?	Nothing.	
Symptoms associated	17 **Heartburn?**	Sometimes.	
	18 **Nausea or vomiting?**	I feel like vomiting.	
	19 **Diarrhea or constipation?**	No.	
	20 **Fever or chills?**	I feel hot when I get the pain.	
	21 **Difficulty breathing or cough?**	No.	
Social Hx	22 What is your **diet** like?	I'm on the road and eat a lot of fast food.	
	23 Changes to the diet, foods left out, etc.?	No.	
	24 Do you **smoke**?	No.	
	25 Do you drink **alcohol**?	A little.	
	26 **How much** do you drink?	A couple of beers a week.	
	27 What is your **occupation**?	I'm a FedEx driver.	
Medical Hx	28 Do you have any medical conditions?	I had about a year ago.	
Allergies	29 Do you have any allergies?	No.	
Surg Hx	30 Have you had any surgeries?	I had a C-section with the baby.	
Hosp Hx	31 Have you ever been hospitalized?	Just the baby.	
Family Hx	32 Medical conditions that run in the family?	Lung problems, but they were smokers.	
	33 Family members/contacts with same symptoms?	No.	
Menstrual Hx	34 When was the **FDLMP**?	I haven't had one since I had the baby.	
Medications	35 Are you on any **medications**?	Just birth control pills.	

Physical Examination ✓

	36	Informs patient that the physical exam is to begin and asks permission.	
	37	Rewashes hands before touching patient if candidate has recontaminated them.	
General	38	Assesses for distress and position of comfort.	**Flexes toward and holds RUQ**
Eyes	39	Inspection	**No icterus**
Respiratory	40	Auscultation performed on bare skin	**Faint crackles in RLL, otherwise CTA**
	41	Through complete inspiration and expiration	
	42	Symmetrically	
	43	At least 2 anterior levels, 1 lateral, and 3 posterior	
Cardiac	44	Auscultation performed on bare skin	**RR without murmurs, rubs, gallops**
	45	Areas: aortic, pulmonic, tricuspid, and mitral	
Abdomen	46	Helps patient to supine position.	
	47	Drapes lower extremities with sheet.	
	48	Inspection	**Moderately obese**
	49	Auscultation prior to palpation	**Hyperactive bowel sounds**
	50	Palpation	**Grimaces greatest in RUQ**
	51	Percussion	**Tympanic in the left upper quad**
	52	Special tests: Rebound, Rigidity, Guarding	**Guarding of the RUQ only**
	53	Murphy's exam	**Positive**
Rectal	54	Advises patient that rectal exam is recommended.	**Not performed on SP**
Assessment	55	Presents patient with a proposed diagnosis.	**Cholelithiasis**
Plan	56	MTHR: Antibiotics, labs, imaging, pain control after surgical consult	
(MOTHRR)	57	Advises admission and surgical evaluation.	
	58	Thanks the patient and asks if there are any questions.	

Humanistic Evaluation Y/N

Did the candidate present in a self-caring manner (e.g., hair control, clothing, cleanliness, aroma, etc.)?	
Did the candidate make periodic eye contact?	
Was the candidate's language clear and EASY to understand?	
Did the candidate have any substance in his or her mouth during the session?	
Did the candidate exhibit body language that would make you feel the candidate was communicating with you?	
Was the candidate enthusiastic?	
Did the candidate exhibit pride in his or her efforts?	
Did the candidate make any comment regarding your lifestyle (e.g., your work, family, activities, etc.)?	
Did the candidate express any humanistic statement recognizing your concerns?	
Did the candidate explain the medical problem and offer you a possible diagnosis?	
Did the candidate suggest a treatment plan that you could understand?	
Did the candidate inquire whether you might want to consult with family members or others about your visit?	
Did the candidate present as if he or she were a competent interviewer?	
Did the candidate ask you if you had any questions?	
Did the candidate thank you?	

Case 34

Patient Name:	Cal Furtz
Clinical Setting:	Family Practice Office
CC:	A 69 y/o male presents for leg pain.

Vital Signs

Blood pressure:	122/68
Respirations:	16 per minute
Temperature:	96.8°F
Pulse:	80 bpm
Weight:	186 lbs
Height:	5' 11"

NOTES:

Subjective

Objective

Assessment

Plan

CC: A 69 y/o male presents for leg pain.

History			✓
	1	Introduces self and explains role of provider.	
	2	Properly washes hands before touching the patient (15-sec wash and turns off with towel).	
	3	Opening question: What brings you in today?	My leg hurts.	
Chronology/ Onset	4	**When** did this start?	Quite a while ago, maybe 6 months.	
	5	Did you ever have this **before**?	Not before then.	
	6	**How often** does it happen?	Nearly every day.	
	7	Are you **doing anything** when it happens?	It happens when I walk.	
	8	**How far** can you walk before it happens?	Only about a block or so.	
	9	Does it come on **suddenly** or **gradually**?	Sort of gradually.	
Description	10	**Where** is the pain?	It's in my left calf.	
	11	Does it **radiate/go** anywhere?	No.	
	12	What does it **feel like**?	It feels tired and then cramps.	
Intensity	13	**How bad** is the pain on a scale from 0 to 10?	It goes as high as a 7.	
Exacerbation	14	Does anything make it **worse**?	Walking.	
Remission	15	What makes it **better**?	It goes away in a minute or two if I rest.	
Symptoms associated	16	**Hair loss on the leg?**	I haven't noticed.	
	17	**Weakness?**	Just in that calf.	
	18	**Numbness or tingling?**	No.	
	19	**Chest pain or shortness of breath?**	No.	
Social Hx	20	What does your **diet** look like?	I'm a meat and potatoes guy.	
(FED TACOS)	21	Do you **exercise**?	Just the walking.	
	22	Do you **smoke**?	A little.	
	23	**How much** a day?	About a half pack.	
	24	**How many years?**	About 30 or so.	
	25	Do you drink **alcohol**?	No.	
	26	Do you drink **caffeine**?	I drink a pot of coffee a day.	
	27	**Occupation?**	I'm an author.	
Medical Hx	28	Do you have any medical conditions?	I have high blood pressure.	
Allergies	29	Do you have any allergies?	No.	
Surg Hx	30	Have you had any surgeries?	None.	
Hosp Hx	31	Have you ever been hospitalized?	No.	
Family Hx	32	Medical conditions that run in the family?	A little blood pressure and sugar.	
Medications	33	Are you on any medications?	Hydrochlorothiazide.	
	34	How many pills a day?	One in the morning and one at night.	
	35	How many milligrams?	50 mg.	

Physical Examination ✓

	36	Informs patient that the physical exam is to begin and asks permission.		
	37	Rewashes hands before touching patient if candidate has recontaminated them.		
Neck	38	Auscultates for carotid bruit bilaterally.	**No bruits**	
Cardiac	39	Auscultation performed on bare skin	**Reg rhythm w/o murmur, rub, or gallop**	
	40	Areas: aortic, pulmonic, tricuspid, and mitral		
Respiratory	41	Auscultation performed on bare skin	**Clear to auscultation**	
	42	Through complete inspiration and expiration		
	43	Symmetrically		
	44	At least 2 anterior levels, 1 lateral, and 3 posterior		
Abdomen	45	Helps patient to supine position.		
	46	Covers lower extremities with a sheet during the exam.		
	47	Inspection: Properly exposes the abdomen	**No masses**	
	48	Auscultation prior to palpation	**NABS without bruit**	
	49	Palpation of size of abdominal aorta	**No pulsatile masses**	
Extremity	50	Inspection: Exposes lower extremities by raising sheet		
	51	Palpates bilaterally: Femoral arteries	**Femoral arteries 2/4 bilaterally**	
Vascular	52	Popliteal arteries	**Unable to be detected**	
	53	Dorsalis pedis and posterior tibialis	**R 2/4 DP and PT, Left not detected**	
Assessment	54	Presents patient with a proposed diagnosis.	**Peripheral arterial disease**	
Plan	55	MTHR: Aspirin, ankle/brachial index, labs, smoking cessation, exercises, referral		
(MOTHRR)	56	Devises and explains a follow-up plan with the patient.		
	57	Thanks the patient and asks if there are any questions.		

Humanistic Evaluation Y/N

Did the candidate present in a self-caring manner (e.g., hair control, clothing, cleanliness, aroma, etc.)?	
Did the candidate make periodic eye contact?	
Was the candidate's language clear and EASY to understand?	
Did the candidate have any substance in his or her mouth during the session?	
Did the candidate exhibit body language that would make you feel the candidate was communicating with you?	
Was the candidate enthusiastic?	
Did the candidate exhibit pride in his or her efforts?	
Did the candidate make any comment regarding your lifestyle (e.g., your work, family, activities, etc.)?	
Did the candidate express any humanistic statement recognizing your concerns?	
Did the candidate explain the medical problem and offer you a possible diagnosis?	
Did the candidate suggest a treatment plan that you could understand?	
Did the candidate inquire whether you might want to consult with family members or others about your visit?	
Did the candidate present as if he or she were a competent interviewer?	
Did the candidate ask you if you had any questions?	
Did the candidate thank you?	

Case 35

Patient Name:	Crystal Ulrich
Clinical Setting:	Urgent Care
CC:	A 54 y/o female presents with foot pain.

Vital Signs

Blood pressure:	158/92
Respirations:	12 per minute
Temperature:	99.0°F
Pulse:	92 bpm
Weight:	155 lbs
Height:	5'5"

NOTES:

Subjective

Objective

Assessment

Plan

CC: A 54 y/o female presents with foot pain.

	History		✓
	1 Introduces self and explains role of provider.		
	2 Properly washes hands before touching the patient (15-sec wash and turns off with towel).		
	3 Opening question: What brings you in today?	My foot is killing me.	
Chronology/ Onset	4 **When** did it start?	It woke me up out of dead sleep last night.	
	5 Did you ever have this **before**?	Once, last year, but it only lasted a day.	
	6 How was it **treated**?	I just took a couple ibuprofen.	
	7 Was there any **trauma/new activity**?	Not that I can think of.	
Description	8 **Describe** the pain.	It feels like it is on fire.	
	9 **Where** is the pain?	It's all in my right big toe.	
	10 Does is **radiate/go anywhere**?	No.	
Intensity	11 **Intensity** on a scale of 1 to 10?	I'd say it's at least an 8.	
Exacerbation	12 What makes it **worse**?	Touching it. Even the sheet hurts it.	
Remission	13 What makes it **better**?	I tried some ibuprofen.	
	14 **How much** did you take?	I took it twice.	
	15 **How much** each time?	600 mg, I think.	
Symptoms associated	16 Any **swelling**?	Yes, a little.	
	17 Any **redness**?	Yes, a lot.	
	18 Any **increased heat**?	Yes, it's hot.	
	19 Any **fever or chills**?	Maybe a little.	
	20 Are you under any **stress**?	No more than usual.	
Social Hx	21 How does your **diet** look?	Probably not as good as it could.	
(FED TACOS)	22 Do you **exercise**?	I walk a couple miles a couple days a week.	
	23 Do you use **tobacco**?	No.	
	24 Do you drink **alcohol**?	Yes.	
	25 How much a day?	Oh, a couple glasses of wine with dinner.	
	26 What is your **occupation**?	I'm a nurse.	
Medical Hx	27 Do you have any medical conditions?	I have high blood pressure.	
Allergies	28 Do you have any allergies?	No.	
Surgical Hx	29 Have you had any surgeries?	I just had my gallbladder out last week.	
	30 How did the surgery go/pain?	Really good. It was laparoscopic. No pain.	
Hosp Hx	31 Have you ever been hospitalized?	Just the gallbladder, and when I had my kids.	
Family Hx	32 Medical conditions that run in the family?	There is some gout in the family.	
Medications	33 Are you on any medications?	I just started a new water pill.	
	34 Do you know the name?	Hydrochlorothiazide.	
	35 When did you start it?	Last week.	

Physical Examination ✓

	36	Informs patient that the physical exam is to begin and asks permission.	
	37	Rewashes hands before touching patient if candidate has recontaminated them.	
General	38	Assesses for distress from pain.	**No grimace while sitting**
Vitals	39	Repeats BP with correct technique.	**BP 146/86**
	40	Appropriate size cuff	
	41	Applied correctly placing cuff on bare arm	
MS	42	Covers patient with sheet, lifting to examine.	
	43	Inspection bilateral feet/ankles	**R foot erythema around 1st MTP joint**
	44	Range of motion	**Ankles full AROM, painful R toe flexion**
	45	Palpation for warmth	**Increase warmth at 1st MTP**
	46	Tenderness	**Exquisitely tender to light palpation**
	47	Bilateral peripheral pulses	**Dorsalis pedis/post tibialis 2/4 b/l**
Respiratory	48	Auscultation performed on bare skin	**Clear to auscultation**
	49	Through complete inspiration and expiration	
	50	Symmetrically	
	51	At least 2 anterior levels, 1 lateral, and 3 posterior	
Cardiac	52	Auscultation performed on bare skin	**RR without murmurs, rubs, gallops**
	53	Areas: aortic, pulmonic, tricuspid, and mitral	
Assessment	54	Presents patient with a proposed diagnosis.	**Acute gout**
Plan	55	MTHR: Anti-inflammatory, BP med change, labs, holistic (RICE), diet/alcohol modification	
(MOTHRR)	56	Explains and offers OMM.	
	57	Performs OMM appropriately (no HVLA).	
	58	Return plan: Devises and explains a follow-up plan with the patient.	
	59	Thanks the patient and asks if there are any questions.	

Humanistic Evaluation Y/N

Did the candidate present in a self-caring manner (e.g., hair control, clothing, cleanliness, aroma, etc.)?	
Did the candidate make periodic eye contact?	
Was the candidate's language clear and EASY to understand?	
Did the candidate have any substance in his or her mouth during the session?	
Did the candidate exhibit body language that would make you feel the candidate was communicating with you?	
Was the candidate enthusiastic?	
Did the candidate exhibit pride in his or her efforts?	
Did the candidate make any comment regarding your lifestyle (e.g., your work, family, activities, etc.)?	
Did the candidate express any humanistic statement recognizing your concerns?	
Did the candidate explain the medical problem and offer you a possible diagnosis?	
Did the candidate suggest a treatment plan that you could understand?	
Did the candidate inquire whether you might want to consult with family members or others about your visit?	
Did the candidate present as if he or she were a competent interviewer?	
Did the candidate ask you if you had any questions?	
Did the candidate thank you?	

Patient Name: Tom A. Gaine
Clinical Setting: Family Practice Outpatient Office Visit
CC: A 76 y/o male presents with hearing loss.

Vital Signs
Blood pressure: 138/72
Respirations: 12 per minute
Temperature: 97.2°F
Pulse: 60 bpm
Weight: 152 lbs
Height: 5'9"

NOTES:

Subjective

Objective

Assessment

Plan

CC: A 76 y/o male presents with hearing loss.

History				✓
	1	Introduces self and explains role of provider.		
	2	Properly washes hands before touching the patient (15-sec wash and turns off with towel).		
	3	Opening question: What brings you in today?	Something is wrong with my hearing.	
Chronology/ Onset	4	**When** did it first **start**?	A couple a months.	
	5	Did this ever happen **before**?	No.	
	6	Has it **changed** in any way?	It's just getting worse.	
Description	7	**Which** ear?	I can't hear out of my right ear.	
	8	Please give examples of **what** can't be heard.	I can't hear my daughter or grandkids.	
Exacerbation	9	What makes it **worse**?	It's worse with a lot of background noise.	
Remission	10	What makes it **better**?	Nothing.	
Symptoms associated	11	Any **ringing** in the ears?	Yes, a little bit.	
	12	Any **dizziness**?	No.	
	13	**Pain**?	A little.	
	14	On a **scale** from 1 to 10, how painful is it?	About a 2.	
	15	**Discharge?**	No.	
	16	**Colds/runny nose/sore throat?**	A little clear runny nose.	
	17	Any **fever/chills**?	No.	
	18	Any **trauma**?	No.	
Social Hx	19	Do you use **tobacco**?	No.	
(FED TACOS)	20	Do you drink **alcohol**?	No.	
	21	What is your **occupation**?	I retired from the steel mill. It was loud.	
Medical Hx	22	Do you have any medical conditions?	The only thing I've got is arthritis.	
Allergies	23	Do you have any allergies?	Just pollens, especially this time of year.	
Surg Hx	24	Have you had any surgeries?	No.	
Hosp Hx	25	Have you ever been hospitalized?	No.	
Family Hx	26	Medical conditions that run in the family?	Just the arthritis.	
Medications	27	Are you on any medications?	I take aspirin a couple times a day.	
	28	How many **milligrams**?	Two extra strengths is all I know.	
	29	How many **times a day**?	Three to 4 times a day.	

Physical Examination ✓

	30	Informs patient that the physical exam is to begin and asks permission.	
	31	Rewashes hands before touching patient if candidate has recontaminated them.	
Ear	32	Inspection	**No deformity, exudate**
	33	Asks for pain: Retracts pinna/depresses tragus.	**No pain with technique**
	34	Performs otoscopic examination.	
	35	Inverts scope and distends finger.	
	36	Performs screening hearing test.	**Reduced hearing in the right ear**
	37	Weber test: Tuning fork to middle of head	**Lateralized to the Left**
	38	Rhinne test: Tuning fork behind ear, then in front	**AC > BC bilaterally**
Nose	39	Inspection	**Nasal mucosal pale with clear exudate**
Throat	40	Inspection	**No erythema or exudate**
Lymph	41	Palpation	**No lymphadenopathy**
Respiratory	42	Auscultation performed on bare skin	**Clear to auscultation**
	43	Through complete inspiration and expiration	
	44	Symmetrically	
	45	At least 2 anterior levels, 1 lateral, and 3 posterior	
Cardiac	46	Auscultation performed on bare skin	**RR without murmurs, rubs, or gallops**
	47	Areas: aortic, pulmonic, tricuspid, and mitral	
Assessment	48	Presents patient with a proposed diagnosis.	**Sensorineural hearing loss, ASA toxicity**
Plan	49	MTHR: NSAID change, hearing test, referral	
(MOTHRR)	50	Return plan: Devises and explains a follow-up plan with the patient.	
	51	Thanks the patient and asks if there are any questions.	

Humanistic Evaluation Y/N

Did the candidate present in a self-caring manner (e.g., hair control, clothing, cleanliness, aroma, etc.)?	
Did the candidate make periodic eye contact?	
Was the candidate's language clear and EASY to understand?	
Did the candidate have any substance in his or her mouth during the session?	
Did the candidate exhibit body language that would make you feel the candidate was communicating with you?	
Was the candidate enthusiastic?	
Did the candidate exhibit pride in his or her efforts?	
Did the candidate make any comment regarding your lifestyle (e.g., your work, family, activities, etc.)?	
Did the candidate express any humanistic statement recognizing your concerns?	
Did the candidate explain the medical problem and offer you a possible diagnosis?	
Did the candidate suggest a treatment plan that you could understand?	
Did the candidate inquire whether you might want to consult with family members or others about your visit?	
Did the candidate present as if he or she were a competent interviewer?	
Did the candidate ask you if you had any questions?	
Did the candidate thank you?	

Case 37

Patient Name:	Buddy Urn
Clinical Setting:	Outpatient Primary Care Visit
CC:	A 69 y/o male presents to the office with hematuria.

Vital Signs

Blood pressure:	126/68
Respirations:	12 per minute
Temperature:	98.8°F
Pulse:	76 bpm
Weight:	173 lbs
Height:	6' 1"

NOTES:

Subjective

Objective

Assessment

Plan

CC: A 69 y/o male presents to the office with hematuria.

History			✓
	1 Introduces self and explains role of provider.		
	2 Properly washes hands before touching the patient (15-sec wash and turns off with towel).		
	3 Opening question: What brings you in today?	There is blood in my urine.	
Chronology/ Onset	4 When did it **start**?	Last night.	
	5 Did you ever have this **before**?	Yes.	
	6 **When**?	It's just been a little pink the last month.	
Description	7 **Describe** the urine.	It's pure red now, with some clots.	
Remittance	8 Anything make it **better**?	I tried to drink more, but it didn't work.	
Symptoms associated	9 Any **trauma/overexercising**?	No.	
	10 **Fever or chills**?	No.	
	11 **Pain**?	No. Nothing hurts at all.	
	12 **Weight loss** or **gain**?	No.	
	13 **Penile discharge**?	No.	
	14 **Dysuria**?	Just a little bit at the start.	
	15 **Hesitancy**?	Yes, I stand there for a while.	
	16 **Frequency**?	Yes. I get up five times a night.	
	17 **Urgency**?	Sometimes.	
Social Hx	18 Do you **smoke**?	No, I quit 5 years ago.	
	19 **How much** before that?	Two packs a day.	
	20 **How many years**?	Since I was 18.	
	21 Do you **drink**?	Yes.	
	22 **How much** a day?	Two beers, once or twice a month.	
	23 What is your **occupation**?	I'm a sales manager.	
Medical Hx	24 Do you have any medical conditions?	Atrial fibrillation.	
Allergies	25 Do you have any allergies?	Yes. Hydrochlorothiazide.	
	26 What is the **reaction**?	My sodium dropped real low.	
Surg Hx	27 Have you had any surgeries?	I had some prostate biopsies last month.	
	28 **Why**?	I had a nodule, but the biopsies were negative.	
Hosp Hx	29 Have you ever been hospitalized?	When I first had the A-fib.	
Family Hx	30 Medical conditions that run in the family?	Some high blood pressure.	
Medications	31 Are you on any medications?	Coumadin.	
	32 How many milligrams a day?	10 mg once a day.	

Physical Examination ✓

	33	Informs patient that the physical exam is to begin and asks permission.	
	34	Rewashes hands before touching patient if candidate has recontaminated them.	
General	35	General assessment	**Alert, no apparent distress**
	36	Position of comfort	
Respiratory	37	Auscultation performed on bare skin	**Clear to auscultation**
	38	Through complete inspiration and expiration	
	39	Symmetrically	
	40	At least 2 anterior levels, 1 lateral, and 3 posterior	
Cardiac	41	Auscultation performed on bare skin	**Irreg w/o murmur, rub, or gallop**
	42	Areas: aortic, pulmonic, tricuspid, and mitral	
Abdominal	43	Helps patient to supine position.	
	44	Drapes lower extremities with sheet.	
	45	Inspection: Properly exposes the abdomen	**Rounded**
	46	Auscultation prior to palpation	**Normoactive bowel sounds, no bruits**
	47	Percussion: Four quadrants	**Superpubic dullness**
	48	Palpation watching facial expression	**Bladder enlargement with tenderness**
CVA	49	CVA tenderness	**Negative**
Genital	50	Advises SP genital exam recommended.	**Does NOT perform exam**
Rectal	51	Advises SP rectal exam recommended.	**Does NOT perform exam**
Assessment	52	Presents patient with a proposed diagnosis.	**Hematuria (BPH vs. UTI, r/o mass)**
Plan	53	MTHR: UA, labs, antibiotics if appropriate, imaging, referral	
(MOTHRR)	54	Return plan: Devises and explains a follow-up plan with the patient.	
	55	Thanks the patient and asks if there are any questions.	

Humanistic Evaluation Y/N

Did the candidate present in a self-caring manner (e.g., hair control, clothing, cleanliness, aroma, etc.)?	
Did the candidate make periodic eye contact?	
Was the candidate's language clear and EASY to understand?	
Did the candidate have any substance in his or her mouth during the session?	
Did the candidate exhibit body language that would make you feel the candidate was communicating with you?	
Was the candidate enthusiastic?	
Did the candidate exhibit pride in his or her efforts?	
Did the candidate make any comment regarding your lifestyle (e.g., your work, family, activities, etc.)?	
Did the candidate express any humanistic statement recognizing your concerns?	
Did the candidate explain the medical problem and offer you a possible diagnosis?	
Did the candidate suggest a treatment plan that you could understand?	
Did the candidate inquire whether you might want to consult with family members or others about your visit?	
Did the candidate present as if he or she were a competent interviewer?	
Did the candidate ask you if you had any questions?	
Did the candidate thank you?	

Case 38

Patient Name: Patricia Pfodz
Clinical Setting: Family Practice Office
CC: A 53 y/o female presents for evaluation of cholesterol.

Vital Signs
Blood pressure: 142/84
Respirations: 16 per minute
Temperature: 96.8°F
Pulse: 74 bpm
Weight: 169 lbs
Height: 5'3"

NOTES:

Subjective

Objective

Assessment

Plan

CC: A 53 y/o female presents for evaluation of cholesterol.

		History		✓
	1	Introduces self and explains role of provider.		
	2	Properly washes hands before touching the patient (15-sec wash and turns off with towel).		
	3	Opening question: What brings you in today?	My church checked our cholesterol and told me to see a doctor.	
Chronology/ Onset	4	**When** were you told that?	A couple of weeks ago.	
	5	Did you ever have this **before**?	No.	
Intensity	6	**How high** was it?	My total was 269.	
	7	Do you know your **HDL and LDL**?	No, I don't know.	
Symptoms associated	8	Do you have any **chest pain**?	No.	
	9	**Shortness of breath/dyspnea on exertion**?	Yes. I get short of breath.	
	10	When?	When I exert myself.	
	11	**How far** can you walk/climb stairs?	About 3 blocks/2 flights of stairs.	
	12	**Weakness or paresthesia**?	No.	
	13	**Slurred speech or difficulty swallowing**?	No.	
	14	**Pain in calves when walking** (claudication)?	No.	
Social Hx	15	What does your **diet** look like?	Seafood . . . whatever food I see, I eat.	
(FED TACOS)	16	Do you **exercise**?	I walk the grocery aisles.	
	17	Do you **smoke**?	No. I quit 10 years ago.	
	18	**How much** did you smoke a day?	About a half pack a day.	
	19	**How long** had you been smoking?	About 20 years.	
	20	Do you drink **alcohol**?	Only a glass of wine once a month or so.	
	21	What is your **occupation**?	I'm an editor.	
Medical Hx	22	Do you have any medical conditions?	I get gout now and then.	
Allergies	23	Do you have any allergies?	Yes.	
	24	What are you allergic to?	Aspirin upsets my stomach.	
Surg Hx	25	Have you had any surgeries?	No.	
Hosp Hx	26	Have you ever been hospitalized?	No.	
Family Hx	27	Medical conditions that run in the family?	Dad had a heart attack. Mom had a stroke.	
Medications	28	Are you on any medications?	I take allopurinol every day.	
	29	How many **milligrams**?	I'm not sure. Sorry.	
	30	How many **times a day**?	Just once.	

Physical Examination ✓

	31	Informs patient that the physical exam is to begin and asks permission.	
	32	Rewashes hands before touching patient if candidate has recontaminated them.	
Vitals	33	Repeats BP with correct technique.	**BP 156/86**
	34	Appropriate size cuff	
	35	Applied correctly placing cuff on bare arm	
Skin	36	Inspection	**No lesions, xanthomas, striae**
Neck	37	Auscultation	**No bruit**
	38	Palpate	**No thyromegaly**
Cardiac	39	Auscultation performed on bare skin	**Reg rhythm w/o murmur, rub, or gallop**
	40	Areas: aortic, pulmonic, tricuspid, and mitral	
	41	Palpation for PMI	**5th ICS midclavicular line**
Respiratory	42	Auscultation performed on bare skin	**Clear to auscultation**
	43	Through complete inspiration and expiration	
	44	Symmetrically	
	45	At least 2 anterior levels, 1 lateral, and 3 posterior	
Abdominal	46	Helps patient with position changes.	
	47	Covers lower extremities with a sheet during the exam.	
	48	Inspection: Properly exposes the abdomen	**No masses**
	49	Auscultation prior to palpation	**NABS without bruit**
	50	Palpation of size of abdominal aorta	**No pulsatile masses**
Vascular	51	Palpation	**Dorsalis pedis/post tibialis 2/4 b/l**
Extremities	52	Inspection	**No edema**
Assessment	53	Presents patient with a proposed diagnosis.	**Hyperlipidemia**
Plan	54	MTHR: Behavioral modification, patient education, ECG, labs	
(MOTHRR)	55	Return plan: Devises and explains a follow-up plan with the patient.	
	56	Thanks the patient and asks if there are any questions.	

Humanistic Evaluation Y/N

Did the candidate present in a self-caring manner (e.g., hair control, clothing, cleanliness, aroma, etc.)?	
Did the candidate make periodic eye contact?	
Was the candidate's language clear and EASY to understand?	
Did the candidate have any substance in his or her mouth during the session?	
Did the candidate exhibit body language that would make you feel the candidate was communicating with you?	
Was the candidate enthusiastic?	
Did the candidate exhibit pride in his or her efforts?	
Did the candidate make any comment regarding your lifestyle (e.g., your work, family, activities, etc.)?	
Did the candidate express any humanistic statement recognizing your concerns?	
Did the candidate explain the medical problem and offer you a possible diagnosis?	
Did the candidate suggest a treatment plan that you could understand?	
Did the candidate inquire whether you might want to consult with family members or others about your visit?	
Did the candidate present as if he or she were a competent interviewer?	
Did the candidate ask you if you had any questions?	
Did the candidate thank you?	

Case 39

Patient Name: Tracy Hart
Clinical Setting: Family Practice Outpatient Office Visit
CC: A 15 y/o female presents with palpitations.

Vital Signs
Blood pressure: 112/60
Respirations: 12 per minute
Temperature: 99°F
Pulse: 128 bpm regular
Weight: 110 lbs
Height: 5'8"

NOTES:

Subjective

Objective

Assessment

Plan

CC: A 15 y/o female presents with palpitations.

History			✓
	1	Introduces self and explains role of provider.	
	2	Properly washes hands before touching the patient (15-sec wash and turns off with towel).	
	3	Opening question: What brings you in today?	My heart's been racing.	
Chronology/ Onset	4	When did it **start**?	A couple of weeks ago.	
	5	What were you **doing when it occurred**?	Maybe riding bikes.	
	6	Have you ever had this **before**?	I don't think so.	
	7	Did it come on **suddenly** or **gradually**?	I'd say gradually.	
Description/	8	Is it **constant** or does it **come and go**?	It's constant.	
Duration	9	How **fast** does it go?	I didn't check.	
Exacerbation	10	Does anything make it **worse**?	It gets faster when I'm really active.	
Remission	11	Does anything make it **better**?	Not really.	
Symptoms associated	12	**Stress or anxiety?**	Not really.	
	13	**Nervousness?**	Yes	
	14	**Chest pain?**	No.	
	15	**Shortness of breath?**	No.	
	16	**Fever or chills?**	No.	
	17	**Nausea or vomiting?**	No.	
	18	**Weight loss or gain?**	Yes, I've lost 20 pounds in 3 months.	
	19	**Hungry or thirsty?**	Mom says I eat like a horse.	
	20	**Caused yourself to vomit?**	No way.	
	21	**Heat or cold intolerance?**	I sweat a lot.	
	22	**Diarrhea or constipation?**	Not really.	
	23	**Urinary frequency?**	No.	
Social Hx	24	Do you **exercise**?	Just at school in gym.	
(FED TACOS)	25	Do you **smoke**?	No.	
	26	Do you drink **alcohol**?	No.	
	27	Do you use any **drugs**?	Ah, come on, Doc.	
	28	What is your **occupation**?	I just go to school.	
Medical Hx	29	Do you have any medical conditions?	No.	
Allergies	30	Do you have any allergies?	No.	
Surg Hx	31	Have you had any surgeries?	No.	
Hosp Hx	32	Have you ever been hospitalized?	No.	
Family Hx	33	Medical conditions that run in the family?	None that I know of.	
Medications	34	Are you on any medications?	Just Tylenol with my periods.	
Sexual Hx	35	When was the **first day last normal menstrual period**?	About 3 weeks ago.	
	36	Has there been any **change to your periods**?	They used to last 5 days, now 1 or 2.	
	37	Are you **sexually active**?	No way!	

Physical Examination ✓

	38	Informs patient that the physical exam is to begin and asks permission.		
	39	Rewashes hands before touching patient if candidate has recontaminated them.		
General	40	Assesses for **distress**.	**Tremors of hands**	
Vitals	41	Correctly performs vitals if appropriate.	**120 bpm regular rhythm**	
Skin	42	Inspection	**No hair loss. Excoriations of the fingers**	
	43	Palpation	**Smooth skin, silky hair texture, no loss**	
HEENT	44	Inspection	**No exophthalmia or dental erosions**	
Neck	45	Inspection	**Symmetrical, mild thyromegaly**	
	46	Auscultation	**No thyroid bruit**	
	47	Palpation	**Thyromegaly without nodules**	
Cardiac	48	Inspection: Properly exposes the chest	**No heave or visible PMI**	
	49	Auscultation performed on bare skin	**Tachycardia, reg rhythm, accentuated S1**	
	50	Areas: aortic, pulmonic, tricuspid and mitral		
	51	Palpation for PMI.	**PMI 5th ICS 4 cm LSB. No thrills**	
Respiratory	52	Auscultation performed on bare skin	**Clear to auscultation**	
	53	Through complete inspiration and expiration		
	54	Symmetrically		
	55	At least 2 anterior levels, 1 lateral, and 3 posterior		
Abdominal	56	Helps patient with position changes.		
	57	Covers lower extremities with a sheet during the exam.		
	58	Inspection: Properly exposes the abdomen	**Scaphoid. No masses**	
	59	Auscultation prior to palpation	**NABS**	
	60	Palpation	**No masses**	
Assessment	61	Presents patient with a proposed diagnosis.	**Hyperthyroidism**	
Plan	62	MTHR: Lab analysis, beta-blocker if diagnosis confirmed, endocrine consult		
(MOTHRR)	63	Return plan: Devises and explains a follow-up plan with the patient.		
	64	Thanks the patient and asks if there are any questions.		

Humanistic Evaluation Y/N

Did the candidate present in a self-caring manner (e.g., hair control, clothing, cleanliness, aroma, etc.)?	
Did the candidate make periodic eye contact?	
Was the candidate's language clear and EASY to understand?	
Did the candidate have any substance in his or her mouth during the session?	
Did the candidate exhibit body language that would make you feel the candidate was communicating with you?	
Was the candidate enthusiastic?	
Did the candidate exhibit pride in his or her efforts?	
Did the candidate make any comment regarding your lifestyle (e.g., your work, family, activities, etc.)?	
Did the candidate express any humanistic statement recognizing your concerns?	
Did the candidate explain the medical problem and offer you a possible diagnosis?	
Did the candidate suggest a treatment plan that you could understand?	
Did the candidate inquire whether you might want to consult with family members or others about your visit?	
Did the candidate present as if he or she were a competent interviewer?	
Did the candidate ask you if you had any questions?	
Did the candidate thank you?	

Case 40

Patient Name:	Eddie Elbel
Clinical Setting:	Primary Care Outpatient Office Visit
CC:	A 43 y/o male presents c/o arm pain.

Vital Signs

Blood pressure:	146/86
Respirations:	12 per minute
Temperature:	98.8°F
Pulse:	72 bpm
Weight:	175 lbs
Height:	6'1"

NOTES:

Subjective

Objective

Assessment

Plan

CC: A 43 y/o male presents c/o arm pain.

History			✓
	1 Introduces self and explains role of provider.		
	2 Properly washes hands before touching the patient (15-sec wash and turns off with towel).		
	3 Opening question: What brings you in today?	My elbow hurts.	
Chronology/ Onset	4 **When** did it start?	A couple of weeks ago.	
	5 What were you **doing** at the time?	I've been playing a lot of golf.	
	6 Has this ever happened **before**?	Yes.	
	7 **When**?	Last year about the same time.	
	8 **Prior diagnosis/How was it treated?**	I didn't see anyone. It just went away.	
Description	9 **Describe** the pain.	It's sharp.	
	10 **Where** is the pain?	The inside of my right elbow.	
Duration	11 Is it **constant** or does it **come and go**?	I'd say it's there all the time.	
Intensity	12 **Intensity** on a scale of 1 to 10?	About a 5.	
Exacerbation	13 What makes it **worse**?	Swinging the club.	
Remission	14 What makes it **better**?	Ibuprofen helps.	
	15 **How much** did you take?	Three tablets.	
	16 How **often** are you taking them?	Every 8 hours.	
Symptoms associated	17 Any **bruising/redness**?	I don't think so.	
	18 Any **swelling**?	No.	
	19 **Numbness or tingling**?	No.	
Social Hx	20 How does your **diet** look?	I stay off the fats.	
(FED TACOS)	21 Do you **exercise**?	I golf three times a week.	
	22 Do you use **tobacco**?	No.	
	23 Do you drink **alcohol**?	Yes.	
	24 **How much** a day?	We have a couple of beers after golfing.	
	25 What is your **occupation**?	I'm a real estate agent.	
Medical Hx	26 Do you have any medical conditions?	No.	
Allergies	27 Do you have any allergies?	Just some seasonal stuff.	
Surg Hx	28 Have you had any surgeries?	No.	
Hosp Hx	29 Have you ever been hospitalized?	No.	
Family Hx	30 Medical conditions that run in the family?	Nothing really. Dad has some prostate thing.	
Medications	31 Are you on any medications?	Zyrtec.	
	32 How much?	10 mg.	
	33 How many times a day?	Once a day.	

Physical Examination ✓

	34	Informs patient that the physical exam is to begin and asks permission.		
	35	Rewashes hands before touching patient if candidate has recontaminated them.		
Vitals	36	Repeats BP with correct technique.	**BP 146/86**	
	37	Appropriate size cuff		
	38	Applied correctly placing cuff on bare arm		
MS	39	Inspection of elbows bilaterally	**No erythema, ecchymosis, deformity**	
	40	Active ROM b/l elbows	**Full active ROM**	
	41	Palpation of bilateral elbows	**Point tenderness over medial epicondyle**	
Special Testing	42	Wrist flexion against resistance	**Results in pain medial epicondyle**	
Respiratory	43	Auscultation performed on bare skin	**Clear to auscultation**	
	44	Through complete inspiration and expiration		
	45	Symmetrically		
	46	At least 2 anterior levels, 1 lateral, and 3 posterior		
Cardiac	47	Auscultation performed on bare skin	**RR without murmurs, rubs, gallops**	
	48	Areas: aortic, pulmonic, tricuspid, and mitral		
Assessment	49	Presents patient with a proposed diagnosis.	**Medial epicondylitis, elevated BP**	
Plan	50	MTHR: Anti-inflammatory, holistic (RICE), BP education		
(MOTHRR)	51	Explains and offers OMM.		
	52	Performs OMM appropriately (no HVLA).		
	53	Return plan: Devises and explains a follow-up plan with the patient.		
	54	Thanks the patient and asks if there are any questions.		

Humanistic Evaluation Y/N

Did the candidate present in a self-caring manner (e.g., hair control, clothing, cleanliness, aroma, etc.)?	
Did the candidate make periodic eye contact?	
Was the candidate's language clear and EASY to understand?	
Did the candidate have any substance in his or her mouth during the session?	
Did the candidate exhibit body language that would make you feel the candidate was communicating with you?	
Was the candidate enthusiastic?	
Did the candidate exhibit pride in his or her efforts?	
Did the candidate make any comment regarding your lifestyle (e.g., your work, family, activities, etc.)?	
Did the candidate express any humanistic statement recognizing your concerns?	
Did the candidate explain the medical problem and offer you a possible diagnosis?	
Did the candidate suggest a treatment plan that you could understand?	
Did the candidate inquire whether you might want to consult with family members or others about your visit?	
Did the candidate present as if he or she were a competent interviewer?	
Did the candidate ask you if you had any questions?	
Did the candidate thank you?	

Case 41

Patient Name:	Frank Prayn
Clinical Setting:	Emergency Room
CC:	A 28 y/o Caucasian male presents with back pain.

Vital Signs

Blood pressure:	138/85
Respirations:	16 per minute
Temperature:	100.8°F
Pulse:	120 bpm
Weight:	162 lbs
Height:	6' 1"

NOTES:

Subjective

Objective

Assessment

Plan

CC: A 28 y/o Caucasian male presents with back pain.

History				✓
	1	Introduces self and explains role of provider.		
	2	Properly washes hands before touching the patient (15-sec wash and turns off with towel).		
	3	Opening question: What brings you in today?	My back really hurts.	
Chronology/ Onset	4	When did it **start**?	About 2 hours ago.	
	5	What were you **doing**?	I was grocery shopping.	
	6	Did you ever have this **before**?	No.	
Description	7	Was the onset **sudden** or **gradual**?	It was very sudden.	
Duration	8	Is it **continuous** or does it **come and go**?	It's always there, but sometimes it gets a little better, then bad again.	
	9	**Describe** the pain.	Like a huge cramp.	
	10	**Where** is the pain?	*Grabs right lateral lumbar area*	
	11	Does it **radiate** anywhere?	It goes down into my right groin.	
	12	**Where** in the groin?	My right ball.	
Intensity	13	**Intensity** on a scale of 1 to 10?	A 10.	
Exacerbation	14	What makes it **worse**?	I don't think anything.	
Remission	15	What makes it **better**?	Nothing.	
Symptoms associated	16	Do you have any **burning with urination**?	No.	
	17	Do you have any **blood in the urine**?	I haven't seen any.	
	18	**Nausea or vomiting?**	I feel like I'm going to vomit.	
	19	**Fever or chills?**	Yes, I'm hot and sweaty.	
Social Hx	20	Do you **smoke**?	No.	
	21	Do you **drink**?	A little.	
	22	**How much** a day?	One or two beers a week.	
	23	What is your **occupation**?	I'm in grad school.	
Medical Hx	24	Do you have any medical conditions?	No.	
Allergies	25	Do you have any allergies?	Penicillin.	
	26	What is the **reaction**?	I get red and swell up.	
Surg Hx	27	Have you had any surgeries?	No.	
Hosp Hx	28	Have you ever been hospitalized?	No.	
Family Hx	29	Medical conditions that run in the family?	High blood pressure in my Dad.	
Medications	30	Are you on any **medications**?	Just vitamins.	
	31	Which vitamins?	A handful of Vitamin C a day.	
	32	Why do you do that?	To keep the colds away.	

Physical Examination ✓

	33	Informs patient that the physical exam is to begin and asks permission.	
	34	Rewashes hands before touching patient if candidate has recontaminated them.	
Vitals	35	Properly performs repeat pulse.	**Regular rhythm at 120 bpm**
Respiratory	36	Auscultation performed on bare skin	**Clear to auscultation**
	37	Through complete inspiration and expiration	
	38	Symmetrically	
	39	At least 2 anterior levels, 1 lateral, and 3 posterior	
Cardiac	40	Auscultation performed on bare skin	**Reg rhythm w/o murmur, rub, or gallop**
	41	Areas: aortic, pulmonic, tricuspid, and mitral	
Abdominal	42	Helps patient to supine position.	
	43	Drapes lower extremities with sheet.	
	44	Inspection: Properly exposes the abdomen	**Scaphoid**
	45	Auscultation prior to palpation	**Hyperactive bowel sounds**
	46	Palpation watching facial expression	**Tenderness in the right lower quadrant**
	47	Percussion: Four quadrants	**Tympanic in the left upper quad**
Special Testing	48	Rebound, rigidity, Rosving's	**Negative**
CVA	49	CVA tenderness	**Positive**
Genital	50	Advises SP genital exam recommended.	**Does NOT perform exam**
Rectal	51	Advises SP rectal exam recommended.	**Does NOT perform exam**
Assessment	52	Presents patient with a proposed diagnosis.	**Nephrolithiasis**
Plan	53	MTHR: UA, labs, IV fluids, imaging, referral	
(MOTHRR)	54	Advises admission and urology consultation.	
	55	Thanks the patient and asks if there are any questions.	

Humanistic Evaluation   Y/N

Did the candidate present in a self-caring manner (e.g., hair control, clothing, cleanliness, aroma, etc.)?	
Did the candidate make periodic eye contact?	
Was the candidate's language clear and EASY to understand?	
Did the candidate have any substance in his or her mouth during the session?	
Did the candidate exhibit body language that would make you feel the candidate was communicating with you?	
Was the candidate enthusiastic?	
Did the candidate exhibit pride in his or her efforts?	
Did the candidate make any comment regarding your lifestyle (e.g., your work, family, activities, etc.)?	
Did the candidate express any humanistic statement recognizing your concerns?	
Did the candidate explain the medical problem and offer you a possible diagnosis?	
Did the candidate suggest a treatment plan that you could understand?	
Did the candidate inquire whether you might want to consult with family members or others about your visit?	
Did the candidate present as if he or she were a competent interviewer?	
Did the candidate ask you if you had any questions?	
Did the candidate thank you?	

Case 42

Patient Name:	Ima Spectin
Clinical Setting:	Family Practice Outpatient Office Visit
CC:	A 32 y/o female presents, stating, "I think I'm pregnant."

Vital Signs

Blood pressure:	112/58
Respirations:	12 per minute
Temperature:	98.8°F
Pulse:	72 bpm
Weight:	175 lbs
Height:	5'8"

NOTES:

Subjective

Objective

Assessment

Plan

CC: A 32 y/o female presents, stating, "I think I'm pregnant."

History				✓
	1	Introduces self and explains role of provider.		
	2	Properly washes hands before touching the patient (15-sec wash and turns off with towel).		
	3	Opening question: What brings you in today?	I think I'm pregnant.	
Description	4	Why to do you think you are pregnant?	I missed my period.	
Onset/	5	When was the **FDLMP**?	Forty-five days ago.	
Chronology	6	Have you ever **been pregnant before**?	Yes.	
Obstetric hx	7	**How many times?**	Once.	
	8	Did you deliver the baby?	She was born on June 12, 2005.	
	9	Did you carry her to term?	She was a week overdue.	
	10	How much did she weigh?	She weighed 7 pounds, 8 ounces.	
	11	Were there any **complications**?	No.	
	12	Any health problems with her now?	No.	
	13	**Any pregnancies you didn't carry to term?**	Yes.	
	14	Can you tell me about it?	We gave one up when I was 18.	
	15	For adoption?	No, I had an abortion.	
Symptoms associated	16	Do you have any **breast tenderness**?	I have a little soreness.	
	17	**Nausea, vomiting?**	Yes, I feel nauseated a lot.	
	18	**Fatigue?**	Yes.	
	19	Increased **frequency** of **urination**?	No.	
	20	Any **vaginal discharge** or **lesions**?	No.	
Social Hx	21	What is your **diet** like?	I'm a vegetarian.	
(FED TACOS)	22	Do you **exercise**?	I do aerobics 3 or 4 days a week.	
	23	Do you **smoke**?	No.	
	24	Do you drink **alcohol**?	One or two drinks every couple of months.	
	25	Do you drink **caffeine**?	No, I drink decaf.	
	26	What is your **occupation**?	I'm an administrative assistant.	
	27	Do you use any drugs?	No.	
	28	Have you or your partner ever had an **STD?**	No.	
	29	Are you **married**?	Yes.	
	30	Did you plan to have a baby?	No. Not really.	
	31	How do you feel about it?	Surprised but happy.	
	32	How does your husband feel about it?	He's happy. He loves kids.	
Medical Hx	33	Do you have any medical conditions?	No.	
Allergies	34	Do you have any allergies?	No.	
Surg Hx	35	Have you had any surgeries?	No.	
Hosp Hx	36	Have you ever been hospitalized?	Just when I delivered my baby.	
Family Hx	37	Medical conditions that run in the family?	No.	
Medications	38	Are you on any **medications**?	No.	

Physical Examination ✓

	39	Informs patient that the physical exam is to begin and asks permission.	
	40	Rewashes hands before touching patient if candidate has recontaminated them.	
General	41	General assessment	**Alert, no apparent distress**
Integumentary	42	Hair texture	**Dry**
Eyes	43	Inspection	**No conjunctival pallor**
Mouth	44	Inspection	**No periodontal disease**
Respiratory	45	Auscultation performed on bare skin	**Clear to auscultation**
	46	Through complete inspiration and expiration	
	47	Symmetrically	
	48	At least 2 anterior levels, 1 lateral, and 3 posterior	
Cardiac	49	Auscultation performed on bare skin	**RR without murmurs, rubs, gallops**
	50	Areas: aortic, pulmonic, tricuspid, and mitral	
Abdomen	51	Helps patient to supine position.	
	52	Drapes lower extremities with sheet.	
	53	Inspection	**Rounded**
	54	Auscultation prior to palpation	**Normoactive bowel sounds**
	55	Palpation	**Cannot palpate uterus**
Extremities	56	Inspection	**No edema**
Breast	57	Advises SP that breast exam should be performed.	**Does not perform exam**
Genitalia	58	Advises SP that pelvic exam should be performed.	**Does not perform exam**
Assessment	59	Presents patient with at least one diagnosis.	**Fertility planning**
Plan	60	MTHR: Folic acid, office urine pregnancy test, diet, exercise, smoking, labs, referral	
(MOTHRR)	61	Calculates the EDC: Naegele's Rule = FDLNMP + 1 week − 3 months + 1 year.	
	62	Return plan: Devises and explains a follow-up plan including breast and pelvic exams.	
	63	Thanks the patient and asks if there are any questions.	

Humanistic Evaluation Y/N

	Y/N
Did the candidate present in a self-caring manner (e.g., hair control, clothing, cleanliness, aroma, etc.)?	
Did the candidate make periodic eye contact?	
Was the candidate's language clear and EASY to understand?	
Did the candidate have any substance in his or her mouth during the session?	
Did the candidate exhibit body language that would make you feel the candidate was communicating with you?	
Was the candidate enthusiastic?	
Did the candidate exhibit pride in his or her efforts?	
Did the candidate make any comment regarding your lifestyle (e.g., your work, family, activities, etc.)?	
Did the candidate express any humanistic statement recognizing your concerns?	
Did the candidate explain the medical problem and offer you a possible diagnosis?	
Did the candidate suggest a treatment plan that you could understand?	
Did the candidate inquire whether you might want to consult with family members or others about your visit?	
Did the candidate present as if he or she were a competent interviewer?	
Did the candidate ask you if you had any questions?	
Did the candidate thank you?	

Case 43

Patient Name:	Billy Ache
Clinical Setting:	Family Practice Office
CC:	A 49 y/o male presents complaining of abdominal pain.

Vital Signs

Blood pressure:	152/92
Respirations:	16 per minute
Temperature:	98.9°F
Pulse:	92 bpm
Weight:	228 lbs
Height:	5'8"

NOTES:

Subjective

Objective

Assessment

Plan

CC: A 49 y/o male presents complaining of abdominal pain.

History				✓
	1	Introduces self and explains role of provider.		
	2	Properly washes hands before touching the patient (15-sec wash and turns off with towel).		
	3	Opening question: What brings you in today?	I have a pain in my stomach.	
Chronology/ Onset	4	When did it **start**?	A couple of days ago.	
	5	Did you ever have this **before**?	Yes, on and off for a few months.	
	6	What have you **done for it in the past**?	I just take antacids.	
	7	**When** does it happen?	It seems like an hour after I eat.	
Description	8	What does it **feel like**?	A gnawing.	
Duration	9	Is it **continuous** or does it **come and go**?	Continuous.	
	10	**Where** is the pain?	Right here. (*Points to epigastria*)	
	11	Does it **radiate** anywhere?	Not really.	
Intensity	12	**Intensity** on a scale of 1 to 10?	An 8.	
Exacerbation	13	What makes it **worse**?	Eating.	
Remission	14	What makes it **better**?	Antacids help a little.	
Symptoms associated	15	**Heartburn?**	That's what I think it is.	
	16	**Nausea or vomiting?**	No.	
	17	**Diarrhea?**	No.	
	18	**Constipation?**	No.	
	19	**Blood in your stools or dark stools?**	Well, they're pretty black.	
	20	**Fever or chills?**	No.	
Social Hx	21	What does your **diet** look like?	I'm a beer and wings guy.	
(FED TACOS)	22	Do you smoke?	Yes.	
	23	**How much** do you smoke a day?	A pack a day.	
	24	**How long** have you been smoking?	About 30 years.	
	25	Do you drink **alcohol**?	Yes.	
	26	How many drinks a day?	Three to four shots and a couple of beers a day.	
	27	Have you ever wanted to quit drinking?	No. You have to have some fun in life.	
	28	Do you use any **drugs**?	No. I'm not into that.	
	29	What is your **occupation**?	I'm a prison guard.	
Medical Hx	30	Do you have any medical conditions?	No.	
Allergies	31	Do you have any allergies?	No.	
Surg Hx	32	Have you had any surgeries?	No.	
Hosp Hx	33	Have you ever been hospitalized?	No.	
Family Hx	34	Medical conditions that run in the family?	My dad died in a car wreck.	
Medications	35	Are you on any medications?	No.	

Physical Examination ✓

	36	Informs patient that the physical exam is to begin and asks permission.	
	37	Rewashes hands before touching patient if candidate has recontaminated them.	
Vitals	38	Repeats BP with correct technique.	**BP 148/88**
	39	Appropriate size cuff	
	40	Applied correctly placing cuff on bare arm	
General	41	Assesses for **distress**.	*Patient holding epigastria*
HEENT	42	Inspection	**No icterus, conjunctiva pale**
Cardiac	43	Auscultation performed on bare skin	**Reg rhythm w/o murmur, rub, or gallop**
	44	Areas: aortic, pulmonic, tricuspid, and mitral	
	45	Palpation for PMI	**5th ICS 5 cm from left sternal border**
Respiratory	46	Auscultation performed on bare skin	**Clear to auscultation**
	47	Through complete inspiration and expiration	
	48	Symmetrically	
	49	At least 2 anterior levels, 1 lateral, and 3 posterior	
Abdominal	50	Helps patient with position changes.	
	51	Covers lower extremities with a sheet during the exam.	
	52	Inspection: Properly exposes the abdomen	**Central obesity**
	53	Auscultation prior to palpation	**Hyperactive bowel sounds**
	54	Palpation	**Grimaces at epigastria. No masses**
	55	Percussion	**Tympanic in the left upper quad**
Special Tests	56	Rebound, Rigidity, Guarding	**Guarding of the epigastria**
	57	Murphy's exam	**Negative**
Rectal	58	Advises that rectal exam is recommended.	**Not performed on SP**
Assessment	59	Presents patient with a proposed diagnosis.	**Peptic ulcer**
Plan	60	MTHR: H2 blocker or PPI, CBC, liver panel, chem, diet/alcohol education, possible EGD	
(MOTHRR)	61	Return plan: Devises and explains a follow-up plan with the patient.	
	62	Thanks the patient and asks if there are any questions.	

Humanistic Evaluation Y/N

Did the candidate present in a self-caring manner (e.g., hair control, clothing, cleanliness, aroma, etc.)?	
Did the candidate make periodic eye contact?	
Was the candidate's language clear and EASY to understand?	
Did the candidate have any substance in his or her mouth during the session?	
Did the candidate exhibit body language that would make you feel the candidate was communicating with you?	
Was the candidate enthusiastic?	
Did the candidate exhibit pride in his or her efforts?	
Did the candidate make any comment regarding your lifestyle (e.g., your work, family, activities, etc.)?	
Did the candidate express any humanistic statement recognizing your concerns?	
Did the candidate explain the medical problem and offer you a possible diagnosis?	
Did the candidate suggest a treatment plan that you could understand?	
Did the candidate inquire whether you might want to consult with family members or others about your visit?	
Did the candidate present as if he or she were a competent interviewer?	
Did the candidate ask you if you had any questions?	
Did the candidate thank you?	

Case 44

Patient Name: Emma Trippen
Clinical Setting: Primary Care Outpatient Office Visit
CC: A 54 y/o female presents c/o arm pain.

Vital Signs
Blood pressure: 126/76
Respirations: 12 per minute
Temperature: 98.8°F
Pulse: 72 bpm
Weight: 132 lbs
Height: 5'3"

NOTES:

Subjective

Objective

Assessment

Plan

CC: A 54 y/o female presents c/o arm pain.

History				✓
	1	Introduces self and explains role of provider.		
	2	Properly washes hands before touching the patient (15-sec wash and turns off with towel).		
	3	Opening question: What brings you in today?	I hurt my shoulder.	
Onset	4	**When** did you hurt it?	The day before yesterday.	
	5	**How/what** were you **doing** at the time?	I tripped on the sidewalk and landed on my shoulder.	
	6	How has it **changed**?	It just hasn't gotten any better.	
Chronology	7	Has this ever happened **before**?	No.	
	8	**Where** is the pain?	*Touches the left lateral shoulder*	
Description	9	Does it **radiate/go** anywhere?	No.	
	10	**Describe** the pain.	It's throbbing.	
Intensity	11	**Intensity** on a scale of 1 to 10?	About a 5.	
Exacerbation	12	What makes it **worse**?	Moving my arm.	
Remission	13	What makes it **better**?	Ibuprofen helps a little.	
	14	**How much** did you take?	Three tablets.	
	15	How **often** are you taking them?	Every 3 hours.	
Symptoms associated	16	**Bruising/redness?**	Yes. It's bruised.	
	17	**Swelling?**	It was swollen last night.	
	18	**Numbness or tingling?**	No.	
	19	**Range of motion** limitation?	Yes. I can't lift my arm all the way up.	
	20	**Weakness?**	No.	
Social Hx	21	Do you **exercise** using your arm?	I walk every day.	
(FED TACOS)	22	Do you **smoke**?	No.	
	23	Do you drink **alcohol**?	Yes.	
	24	**How much** a day?	A glass of wine with dinner now and then.	
	25	What is your **occupation**?	I'm a teacher.	
	26	When was the **FDLMP**?	I stopped having periods a few years ago.	
Medical Hx	27	Do you have any medical conditions?	No.	
Allergies	28	Do you have any allergies?	Some pollens bother me.	
Surg Hx	29	Have you had any surgeries?	No.	
Hosp Hx	30	Have you ever been hospitalized?	No.	
Family Hx	31	Medical conditions that run in the family?	Diabetes runs in the family.	
Medications	32	Are you on any medications?	Cetirizine.	
	33	How much?	10 mg.	
	34	How many times a day?	Once a day.	

Physical Examination ✓

	35	Informs patient that the physical exam is to begin and asks permission.	
	36	Rewashes hands before touching patient if candidate has recontaminated them.	
Neck	37	Inspection	**Symmetrical**
	38	Active range of motion	**Full AROM**
	39	Palpation	**Nontender to palpation**
Respiratory	40	Auscultation performed on bare skin	**Clear to auscultation**
	41	Through complete inspiration and expiration	
	42	Symmetrically	
	43	At least 2 anterior levels, 1 lateral, and 3 posterior	
Cardiac	44	Auscultation performed on bare skin	**RR without murmurs, rubs, gallops**
	45	Areas: aortic, pulmonic, tricuspid, and mitral	
MS	46	Inspection of shoulders with proper exposure	**Erythema/ecchymosis L post shoulder**
	47	Bilateral comparison	**No boney deformity**
	48	Palpation	**Tenderness at supraspinatus insertion**
	49	Active range of motion	**Unable to abduct beyond 90 degrees**
	50	Passive range of motion	**Pain with adduction beyond 90 degrees**
Special testing	51	Drop arm test	**Cannot hold arm up**
Neurologic	52	Reflexes—b/l upper extremity	**2/4 bicep, triceps, brachioradialis**
Special Testing	53	Arm drop test	**Positive**
Assessment	54	Presents patient with a proposed diagnosis.	**Rotator cuff injury**
Plan	55	MTHR: Pain control (reduce ibuprofen), shoulder X-ray, holistic (RICE), referral	
(MOTHRR)	56	Explains and offers OMM.	
	57	Performs OMM appropriately (no HVLA).	
	58	Return plan: Devises and explains a follow-up plan with the patient.	
	59	Thanks the patient and asks if there are any questions.	

Humanistic Evaluation Y/N

	Y/N
Did the candidate present in a self-caring manner (e.g., hair control, clothing, cleanliness, aroma, etc.)?	
Did the candidate make periodic eye contact?	
Was the candidate's language clear and EASY to understand?	
Did the candidate have any substance in his or her mouth during the session?	
Did the candidate exhibit body language that would make you feel the candidate was communicating with you?	
Was the candidate enthusiastic?	
Did the candidate exhibit pride in his or her efforts?	
Did the candidate make any comment regarding your lifestyle (e.g., your work, family, activities, etc.)?	
Did the candidate express any humanistic statement recognizing your concerns?	
Did the candidate explain the medical problem and offer you a possible diagnosis?	
Did the candidate suggest a treatment plan that you could understand?	
Did the candidate inquire whether you might want to consult with family members or others about your visit?	
Did the candidate present as if he or she were a competent interviewer?	
Did the candidate ask you if you had any questions?	
Did the candidate thank you?	

Case 45

Patient Name:	Fred Train
Clinical Setting:	Primary Care Office Visit
CC:	A 42 y/o obese male complains of excessive fatigue.

Vital Signs

Blood pressure:	165/98
Respirations:	16 per minute
Temperature:	98.0°F
Pulse:	62 bpm
Weight:	355 lbs
Height:	5'11"

NOTES:

Subjective

Objective

Assessment

Plan

CC: A 42 y/o obese male complains of excessive fatigue.

History			✓
	1 Introduces self and explains role of provider.		
	2 Properly washes hands before touching the patient (15-sec wash and turns off with towel).		
	3 Opening question: What brings you in today?	I can't keep my eyes open. I fall asleep at work. I'm going to lose my job.	
Chronology/ Onset	4 **When** did this start?	Oh, it's been years, Doc.	
	5 How has it **changed**?	I fall asleep 3 or 4 times a day.	
Description	6 **Describe** what's been happening.	I'm just tired.	
Intensity	7 Have you ever fallen asleep while driving?	No.	
Exacerbations	8 Does anything make this **worse**?	No.	
Remissions	9 Does anything make this **better**?	No.	
Symptoms associated	10 Do you **snore**?	My wife says I do.	
	11 Does your wife say you ever **stop breathing**?	Yeah, she's said that.	
	12 Do you **wake yourself up**?	Yeah, quite a bit.	
	13 How do you **sleep at night**?	I just don't feel rested when I get up.	
	14 Problems **concentrating**?	Yeah, I can never finish a TV show.	
	15 **Depression**?	Yeah, I'm down, but wouldn't you be?	
	16 **Anxiety or panic attacks?**	No.	
	17 **Heartburn?**	No.	
Social Hx	18 What does your **diet** look like?	I eat too much. I know it.	
(FED TACOS)	19 Do you **exercise**?	No. No, I don't.	
	20 Do you **smoke**?	No.	
	21 Do you drink **alcohol**?	I have a couple of beers a night.	
	22 What is your **occupation**?	I'm an IT guy.	
Medical Hx	23 Do you have any medical conditions?	High blood pressure and low thyroid.	
Allergies	24 Do you have any allergies?	No.	
Surg Hx	25 Have you had any surgeries?	No.	
Hosp Hx	26 Have you ever been hospitalized?	I had pneumonia once.	
	27 **When** was that?	About 5 years ago.	
Family Hx	28 Does anything run in the family?	Heart problems.	
Medications	29 What **medications** are you on?	Atenolol and Synthroid.	
	30 How many **milligrams**?	20 atenolol, and I'm not sure of the other.	
	31 How many **times a day**?	One each.	

Physical Examination ✓

	32	Informs patient that the physical exam is to begin and asks permission.	
	33	Rewashes hands before touching patient if candidate has recontaminated them.	
Vitals	34	Repeats BP with correct technique.	**BP 168/96**
	35	Appropriate size cuff	
	36	Applied correctly placing cuff on bare arm	
General	37	General assessment	**Fatigued appearance, obese**
HEENT	38	Inspection	**Infraorbital venous pooling. Edentulous**
Neck	39	Inspection	**Large, symmetrical without masses**
	40	Palpation	**No masses or thyromegaly**
Cardiac	41	Auscultation performed on bare skin	**Distant. Reg rhythm, S3 w/o murmur**
	42	Areas: aortic, pulmonic, tricuspid, and mitral	
	43	Palpation for PMI	**Cannot be detected**
Respiratory	44	Auscultation performed on bare skin	**Diminished basilar breath sounds**
	45	Through complete inspiration and expiration	**Crackles bilateral lower lobes**
	46	Symmetrically	
Abdomen	47	Inspection, auscultation, palpation order	**Obese, hypoactive bowel sounds**
Neurologic	48	Orientation	**Alert & oriented × 3**
	49	Muscle strength: B/l upper/lower extremities	**5/5 throughout**
	50	Reflexes: Bilateral upper and lower extremities	**1/4 throughout**
Extremities	51	Inspection	**Without pitting**
Assessment	52	Presents patient with a proposed diagnosis.	**Sleep apnea**
Plan	53	MTHR: BP medication adjustment, labs (thyroid), smoking cessation, sleep study, dietitian	
(MOTHRR)	54	Advises admission and cardiac evaluation.	
	55	Return plan: Devises and explains a follow-up plan with the patient.	
	56	Thanks the patient and asks if there are any questions.	

Humanistic Evaluation Y/N

Did the candidate present in a self-caring manner (e.g., hair control, clothing, cleanliness, aroma, etc.)?	
Did the candidate make periodic eye contact?	
Was the candidate's language clear and EASY to understand?	
Did the candidate have any substance in his or her mouth during the session?	
Did the candidate exhibit body language that would make you feel the candidate was communicating with you?	
Was the candidate enthusiastic?	
Did the candidate exhibit pride in his or her efforts?	
Did the candidate make any comment regarding your lifestyle (e.g., your work, family, activities, etc.)?	
Did the candidate express any humanistic statement recognizing your concerns?	
Did the candidate explain the medical problem and offer you a possible diagnosis?	
Did the candidate suggest a treatment plan that you could understand?	
Did the candidate inquire whether you might want to consult with family members or others about your visit?	
Did the candidate present as if he or she were a competent interviewer?	
Did the candidate ask you if you had any questions?	
Did the candidate thank you?	

Case 46

Patient Name:	Ika Chimney
Clinical Setting:	Family Practice Office
CC:	A 38 y/o male presents to quit smoking.

Vital Signs

Blood pressure:	152/86
Respirations:	16 per minute
Temperature:	96.8°F
Pulse:	62 bpm
Weight:	182 lbs
Height:	6' 2"

NOTES:

Subjective

Objective

Assessment

Plan

CC: A 38 y/o male presents to quit smoking.

History				✓
	1	Introduces self and explains role of provider.		
	2	Properly washes hands before touching the patient (15-sec wash and turns off with towel).		
	3	Opening question: What brings you in today?	I really want to quit smoking.	
Chronology/ Onset	4	When did you **start** smoking?	About 20 years ago.	
	5	Have you ever tried to **quit before**?	Yes.	
	6	How long ago was that?	About 2 years ago.	
	7	How long were you able to quit for?	Three months.	
	8	How did you quit?	Just cold turkey.	
	9	What made you start smoking again?	I got laid off and my brother died.	
Intensity	10	**How much** do you smoke a day?	About a pack.	
Symptoms associated	11	Do you have a **cough**?	Yes.	
	12	All the time, or does it come and go?	All the time.	
	13	Are you **bringing anything up** with it?	Yes, especially in the morning.	
	14	What does it look like?	It's thick and yellow.	
	15	**Chest pain?**	No.	
	16	**Shortness of breath?**	Yes.	
	17	Can you go up two flights of stairs w/o SOB? (*or other quantifier*)	Yes, I think so.	
	18	**Weight loss?**	No.	
	19	**Lightheadedness?**	No.	
	20	**Pain in your legs when you walk?**	No.	
	21	**Numbness/tingling, weakness?**	No.	
Social Hx	22	Do you follow any **diet**?	Not really.	
(FED TACOS)	23	Do you **exercise**?	Not really.	
	24	Do you drink **alcohol**?	Maybe a drink or two a month.	
	25	Do you drink **caffeine**?	A couple pops a day.	
	26	Do you use any **drugs**?	No.	
	27	What is your **occupation**?	I work for a plastics company.	
Medical Hx	28	Do you have any medical conditions?	Not so far.	
Allergies	29	Do you have any allergies?	No.	
Surg Hx	30	Have you had any surgeries?	No.	
Hosp Hx	31	Have you ever been hospitalized?	No.	
Family Hx	32	Does anything run in the family?	My dad had a heart attack when he was 50.	
	33	Are you around others who smoke?	My wife does. She should quit, too.	
	34	Past surgeries or hospitalizations?	None.	
Medications	35	Are you on any medications?	No.	

Physical Examination ✓

	36	Informs patient that the physical exam is to begin and asks permission.	
	37	Rewashes hands before touching patient if candidate has recontaminated them.	
Vitals	38	Repeats BP.	**BP 146/76**
	39	Appropriate size cuff	
	40	Applied correctly placing cuff on bare arm	
HEENT	41	Inspection	**No lesions**
Neck	42	Inspection	**Symmetrical without masses**
	43	Auscultation	**No bruit**
Cardiac	44	Inspection: Properly exposes the chest	**No heave or visible PMI**
	45	Auscultation performed on bare skin	**Reg rhythm w/o murmur, rub, or gallop**
	46	Areas: aortic, pulmonic, tricuspid, and mitral	
	47	Palpation for PMI	**5th ICS 4 cm from left sternal border**
Respiratory	48	Auscultation performed on bare skin	**Clear to auscultation**
	49	Through complete inspiration and expiration	
	50	Symmetrically	
	51	At least 2 anterior levels, 1 lateral, and 3 posterior	
Abdominal	52	Helps patient with position changes.	
	53	Covers lower extremities with a sheet during the exam.	
	54	Inspection: Properly exposes the abdomen	**No masses**
	55	Auscultation prior to palpation	**NABS without bruit**
	56	Palpation of size of abdominal aorta	**No pulsatile masses**
Vascular	57	Palpation	**Peripheral pulses 2/4 throughout**
Assessment	58	Presents patient with a proposed diagnosis.	**Tobacco use disorder, elevated BP**
Plan	59	MTHR: Patient education on smoking cessation options, labs, imaging, referral	
(MOTHRR)	60	Return plan: Devises and explains a follow-up plan with bp check.	
	61	Thanks the patient and asks if there are any questions.	

Humanistic Evaluation Y/N

Did the candidate present in a self-caring manner (e.g., hair control, clothing, cleanliness, aroma, etc.)?	
Did the candidate make periodic eye contact?	
Was the candidate's language clear and EASY to understand?	
Did the candidate have any substance in his or her mouth during the session?	
Did the candidate exhibit body language that would make you feel the candidate was communicating with you?	
Was the candidate enthusiastic?	
Did the candidate exhibit pride in his or her efforts?	
Did the candidate make any comment regarding your lifestyle (e.g., your work, family, activities, etc.)?	
Did the candidate express any humanistic statement recognizing your concerns?	
Did the candidate explain the medical problem and offer you a possible diagnosis?	
Did the candidate suggest a treatment plan that you could understand?	
Did the candidate inquire whether you might want to consult with family members or others about your visit?	
Did the candidate present as if he or she were a competent interviewer?	
Did the candidate ask you if you had any questions?	
Did the candidate thank you?	

Case 47

Patient Name:	Jack E. Cartia
Clinical Setting:	Emergency Room
CC:	A 79 y/o male presents for "funny heart beats."

Vital Signs

Blood pressure:	122/68
Respirations:	16 per minute
Temperature:	96.8°F
Pulse:	120 bpm
Weight:	230 lbs
Height:	6' 1"

NOTES:

Subjective

Objective

Assessment

Plan

CC: A 79 y/o male presents for "funny heart beats."

History			✓
	1	Introduces self and explains role of provider.	
	2	Properly washes hands before touching the patient (15-sec wash and turns off with towel).	
	3	Opening question: What brings you in today?	My heart seems to beat funny.
Chronology/ Onset	4	**When** did this start?	Maybe a month or two ago.
	5	Did you ever have this **before**?	No.
	6	**How often** does it happen?	A couple times a day.
	7	Are you **doing anything** when it happens?	Nothing in particular.
	8	Does it come on **suddenly** or **gradually**?	Suddenly, like flipping a switch.
Description	9	Could you **describe "funny"**?	It goes real fast now and then.
Duration	10	**How long does it last** when it happens?	Only a few minutes.
Intensity	11	How **fast** does it go?	I didn't measure it.
Exacerbation	12	Does anything make it **worse**?	Nothing I've noticed.
Remission	13	What makes it **better**?	Not really.
Symptoms associated	14	**Lightheadedness or dizziness?**	No.
	15	**Shortness of breath?**	No.
	16	**Chest pain?**	No.
	17	**Stress or anxiety?**	No.
Social Hx	18	What does your **diet** look like?	Oh, a sandwich and soup does the job.
(FED TACOS)	19	Do you **exercise**?	I'm too old for that.
	20	Do you **smoke**?	A little.
	21	**How much** do you smoke a day?	About a half pack.
	22	**How long** have you been smoking?	A long, long time. I can't remember.
	23	Do you drink **alcohol**?	No.
	24	Do you drink **caffeine**?	I drink a pot of coffee a day.
	25	What is your **occupation**?	I'm an author.
Medical Hx	26	Do you have any medical conditions?	I have high blood pressure.
Allergies	27	Do you have any allergies?	No.
Surg Hx	28	Have you had any surgeries?	None.
Hosp Hx	29	Have you ever been hospitalized?	No.
Family Hx	30	Medical conditions that run in the family?	A little blood pressure and sugar.
Medications	31	Are you on any medications?	Hydrochlorothiazide.
	32	Do you know the doses?	50 mg.
	33	How many times a day do you take each?	One in the morning and one at night.

Physical Examination ✓

	34	Informs patient that the physical exam is to begin and asks permission.	
	35	Rewashes hands before touching patient if candidate has recontaminated them.	
Vitals	36	Correctly repeats the pulse.	**Irregular, at 124 bpm**
Neck	37	Auscultation for carotid bruit	**No bruit**
	38	Palpitation of thyroid	**No thyromegaly**
	39	Asks patient to swallow during palpation.	
Cardiac	40	Inspection: Properly exposes the chest	**No heave or visible PMI**
	41	Auscultation performed on bare skin	**Irreg with 2/6 SEM at aortic area**
	42	Areas: aortic, pulmonic, tricuspid, and mitral	
	43	Palpation for PMI	**Not detected**
Respiratory	44	Auscultation performed on bare skin	**Clear to auscultation**
	45	Through complete inspiration and expiration	
	46	Symmetrically	
	47	At least 2 anterior levels, 1 lateral, and 3 posterior	
Assessment	48	Presents patient with a proposed diagnosis.	**Atrial fibrillation**
Plan	49	MTHR: Anticoagulation, rate control, imaging, ECG, labs, smoking/caffeine cessation, referral	
(MOTHRR)	50	Advises admission and cardiac evaluation.	
	51	Thanks the patient and asks if there are any questions.	

Humanistic Evaluation Y/N

Did the candidate present in a self-caring manner (e.g., hair control, clothing, cleanliness, aroma, etc.)?	
Did the candidate make periodic eye contact?	
Was the candidate's language clear and EASY to understand?	
Did the candidate have any substance in his or her mouth during the session?	
Did the candidate exhibit body language that would make you feel the candidate was communicating with you?	
Was the candidate enthusiastic?	
Did the candidate exhibit pride in his or her efforts?	
Did the candidate make any comment regarding your lifestyle (e.g., your work, family, activities, etc.)?	
Did the candidate express any humanistic statement recognizing your concerns?	
Did the candidate explain the medical problem and offer you a possible diagnosis?	
Did the candidate suggest a treatment plan that you could understand?	
Did the candidate inquire whether you might want to consult with family members or others about your visit?	
Did the candidate present as if he or she were a competent interviewer?	
Did the candidate ask you if you had any questions?	
Did the candidate thank you?	

Case 48

Patient Name:	Mau Ho
Clinical Setting:	Primary Care Office Visit
CC:	A 62 y/o Vietnamese male presents with a cough (daughter is translating).

Vital Signs

Blood pressure:	100/49
Respirations:	24 per minute
Temperature:	101.5°F
Pulse:	110 bpm
Weight:	126 lbs
Height:	5' 2"

NOTES:

Subjective

Objective

Assessment

Plan

CC: A 62 y/o Vietnamese male presents with a cough (daughter is translating).

History			✓
	1 Introduces self and explains role of provider.		
	2 Properly washes hands before touching the patient (15-sec wash and turns off with towel).		
	3 Opening question: What brings you in today?	He doesn't speak English. He has a cough.	
Chronology/ Onset	4 When did it **start**?	He's had it for several weeks.	
	5 Was the onset **sudden** or **gradual**?	Gradual.	
	6 Did he ever have this **before**?	No.	
Description	7 **Describe** the cough.	He coughs all the time.	
	8 Is he **bringing anything up**?	Not much, but there's blood in it.	
Exacerbations	9 Anything make it **worse**?	It can't get any worse.	
Remittance	10 Anything make it **better**?	No.	
Symptoms associated	11 **Shortness of breath?**	Just if he's coughing really hard.	
	12 **Fever or chills?**	Yes, especially at night.	
	13 **Chest pain?**	He complains of his right side hurting.	
	14 **When?**	When he breathes deeply or coughs.	
	15 **Night sweats?**	He wakes up completely soaked.	
	16 **Shortness of breath lying flat?**	No.	
	17 **Swelling** of the extremities?	No.	
	18 **Weight loss?**	Oh, yes. His pants are falling off.	
	19 How much weight?	Twenty pounds.	
	20 Over what period of time?	Maybe 3 months.	
Social Hx	21 Does he **smoke**?	No.	
(FED TACOS)	22 Does he drink **alcohol**?	No	
	23 What is his **occupation**?	He doesn't work now. He was a farmer.	
	24 **Recent travel?**	He came from Vietnam 6 weeks ago.	
Medical Hx	25 Does he have any medical conditions?	He would never see a doctor before.	
Allergies	26 Does he have any allergies?	Not that I know of.	
Surg Hx	27 Has he had any surgeries?	A broken arm once.	
Hosp Hx	28 Has he ever been hospitalized?	Not that I know of.	
Family Hx	29 Medical conditions that run in the family?	I don't know.	
Medications	30 Is he on any medications?	No.	

Physical Examination ✓

	31	Excuses self to retrieve face mask.	
	32	Informs patient that the physical exam is to begin and asks permission.	
	33	Rewashes hands before touching patient if candidate has recontaminated them.	
Vitals	34	Repeats respirations.	**24 breaths per minute**
	35	Repeats pulse.	**110 beats per minute**
General	36	General assessment	**Appears chronically ill/malnourished**
HEENT	37	Inspection: Nasal/buccal mucosa and pharynx	**No exudate or erythema**
Lymphatics	38	Palpation of all regions	**R supraclavicular lymphadenopathy**
Respiratory	39	Inspection: Properly exposes the chest	**Symmetrical rise and fall**
	40	Auscultation performed on bare skin	**Faint apical rales**
	41	Through complete inspiration and expiration	**Guards R side with deep inspiration**
	42	Symmetrically	
	43	At least 2 anterior levels, 1 lateral, and 3 posterior	
	44	Palpation	**Nontender without masses**
	45	Tactile fremitus	**Symmetrical throughout**
Special Tests	46	Egophony, bronchophony, whispered pectoriloquy	**Negative for consolidation**
Cardiac	47	Auscultation performed on bare skin	**RR without murmurs, rubs, or gallop**
	48	Areas: aortic, pulmonic, tricuspid, and mitral	
Assessment	49	Presents patient with a proposed diagnosis.	**Tuberculosis**
Plan	50	MTHR: Referral ID/Department of Health, imaging, PPD placement, sputum cultures, antibiotics, family screening, education	
(MOTHRR)	51	Return plan: Devises and explains a follow-up plan with the patient.	
	52	Thanks the patient and asks if there are any questions.	

Humanistic Evaluation Y/N

Did the candidate present in a self-caring manner (e.g., hair control, clothing, cleanliness, aroma, etc.)?	
Did the candidate make periodic eye contact?	
Was the candidate's language clear and EASY to understand?	
Did the candidate have any substance in his or her mouth during the session?	
Did the candidate exhibit body language that would make you feel the candidate was communicating with you?	
Was the candidate enthusiastic?	
Did the candidate exhibit pride in his or her efforts?	
Did the candidate make any comment regarding your lifestyle (e.g., your work, family, activities, etc.)?	
Did the candidate express any humanistic statement recognizing your concerns?	
Did the candidate explain the medical problem and offer you a possible diagnosis?	
Did the candidate suggest a treatment plan that you could understand?	
Did the candidate inquire whether you might want to consult with family members or others about your visit?	
Did the candidate present as if he or she were a competent interviewer?	
Did the candidate ask you if you had any questions?	
Did the candidate thank you?	

Patient Name: Theodora Sun
Clinical Setting: Family Practice Office
CC: A 32 y/o female presents for "headaches."

Vital Signs
Blood pressure: 108/72
Respirations: 17 per minute
Temperature: 98.6°F
Pulse: 80 bpm
Weight: 145 lbs
Height: 5'7"

NOTES:

Subjective

Objective

Assessment

Plan

CC: A 32 y/o female presents for "headaches."

History			✓
	1	Introduces self and explains role of provider.	
	2	Properly washes hands before touching the patient (15-sec wash and turns off with towel).	
	3	Opening question: What brings you in today?	I've been having headaches	
Chronology/ Onset	4	**When** did this start?	About 2 weeks ago.	
	5	Did you ever have this **before**?	Not really.	
	6	**How often** does it happen?	Almost every day.	
	7	What are you **doing** when it happens?	Usually typing on my computer.	
	8	Does it come on **suddenly** or **gradually**?	Gradually.	
Description	9	Can you **describe the pain**?	It feels like a tight band around my head.	
Duration	10	**How long does it last** when it happens?	Several hours.	
Intensity	11	How severe is it, on a scale from **1 to 10**?	It's a 3 to 5.	
Exacerbation	12	Does anything make it **worse**?	Lack of sleep.	
Remission	13	What makes it **better**?	Ibuprofen or acetaminophen help.	
	14	How much do you take?	Whatever it says on the bottle.	
	15	How often do you take it?	A couple times a day.	
Symptoms associated	16	**Recent cold?**	No.	
	17	**History of migraines?**	No.	
	18	**Nausea or vomiting?**	No.	
	19	**Recent trauma?**	No.	
	20	**Photophobia or phonophobia?**	No.	
	21	**Numbness or tingling?**	No.	
	22	**Visual changes?**	No.	
Social Hx	23	What does your **diet** look like?	I think it's fairly balanced. I avoid sweets.	
(FED TACOS)	24	Do you **exercise**?	Yes, I work out.	
	25	Do you **smoke**?	No.	
	26	Do you drink **alcohol**?	No.	
	27	Do you drink **caffeine**?	I drink a couple energy drinks a week.	
	28	Do you use any **drugs**?	No.	
	29	What is your **occupation**?	Telemarketing.	
Medical Hx	30	Do you have any medical conditions?	No.	
Allergies	31	Do you have any allergies?	No.	
Surgical Hx	32	Have you had any surgeries?	No.	
Hosp Hx	33	Have you ever been hospitalized?	No.	
Family Hx	34	Any medical conditions that run in the family?	Some cholesterol problems.	
Medications	35	Are you on any medications?	No.	

Physical Examination ✓

	36	Informs patient that the physical exam is to begin and asks permission.	
	37	Rewashes hands before touching patient if candidate has recontaminated them.	
Head	38	Inspection	**NCAT without lesions**
	39	Palpation	**Nontender**
Sinuses	40	Palpation, percussion	**Nontender**
Eyes	41	Assesses visual acuity.	**20/20 b/l**
	42	Pupillary reflex—CNII and CNIII	**Intact**
	43	Extraocular motion (CNIII, IV, VI)	**Intact**
	44	Ophthalmoscopic examination	**Cup: disc ratio 1:2 with sharp margins**
Nose	45	Inspection	**No exudate, edema, masses**
Ears	46	Inspection	**TM's gray bilaterally**
Mouth/throat	47	Inspection	**Teeth in good repair, no lesions, moist**
Neck	48	Palpation	**Tissue texture changes T1-4 b/l. C3SrRr. No nuchal rigidity or tenderness**
Respiratory	49	Auscultation performed on bare skin	**Clear to auscultation**
	50	At least 2 anterior levels, 1 lateral, and 3 posterior	
Cardiac	51	Auscultation performed on bare skin	**RR without murmurs, rubs, or gallop**
	52	Areas: aortic, pulmonic, tricuspid, and mitral	
Neurologic	53	Motor strength testing with b/l comparison	**5/5 throughout**
	54	Reflexes	**2/4 throughout**
Assessment	55	Presents patient with a proposed diagnosis.	**Tension HA, cervical somatic dysfunction**
Plan	56	MTHR: Pain relief, ergonomic education, cholesterol screen	
(MOTHRR)	57	Explains and offers OMM.	
	58	Performs OMM appropriately (no HVLA).	
	59	Return plan: Devises and explains a follow-up plan with the patient.	
	60	Thanks the patient and asks if there are any questions.	

Humanistic Evaluation Y/N

Did the candidate present in a self-caring manner (e.g., hair control, clothing, cleanliness, aroma, etc.)?	
Did the candidate make periodic eye contact?	
Was the candidate's language clear and EASY to understand?	
Did the candidate have any substance in his or her mouth during the session?	
Did the candidate exhibit body language that would make you feel the candidate was communicating with you?	
Was the candidate enthusiastic?	
Did the candidate exhibit pride in his or her efforts?	
Did the candidate make any comment regarding your lifestyle (e.g., your work, family, activities, etc.)?	
Did the candidate express any humanistic statement recognizing your concerns?	
Did the candidate explain the medical problem and offer you a possible diagnosis?	
Did the candidate suggest a treatment plan that you could understand?	
Did the candidate inquire whether you might want to consult with family members or others about your visit?	
Did the candidate present as if he or she were a competent interviewer?	
Did the candidate ask you if you had any questions?	
Did the candidate thank you?	

Case 50

Patient Name:	Mary Jo Freqaunty
Clinical Setting:	Primary Care Outpatient Office Visit
CC:	A 68 y/o female presents c/o being up all night going to the bathroom.

Vital Signs

Blood pressure:	118/76
Respirations:	12 per minute
Temperature:	99.9°F
Pulse:	72 bpm
Weight:	120 lbs
Height:	5'4"

NOTES:

Subjective

Objective

Assessment

Plan

CC: A 68 y/o female presents c/o being up all night going to the bathroom.

History				✓
	1	Introduces self and explains role of provider.		
	2	Properly washes hands before touching the patient (15-sec wash and turns off with towel).		
	3	Opening question: What brings you in today?	I'm up all night peeing.	
Onset	4	**When** did this start?	It's been almost a month now.	
Chronology	5	Has this ever happened **before**?	No.	
Intensity	6	**How many times** a night?	At least four or five.	
Exacerbation	7	Does anything make it **worse**?	No.	
Remission	8	What makes it **better**?	Nothing.	
Symptoms associated	9	Increased **thirst**?	No.	
	10	Increased **hunger**?	No.	
	11	**Weight loss?**	No.	
	12	**Fever?**	No.	
	13	**Fatigue?**	Yes, I'm tired but I'm not sleeping.	
	14	**Burning** with urination?	Yes, it burns a little.	
	15	**Pain?**	I feel a pressure in my bladder.	
	16	**Urgency?**	When I have to go, I have to go.	
	17	**Blood** in the urine?	Not that I've seen.	
	18	**Malodor?**	Yes, it smells strong.	
	19	What does the urine **look like**/is it **cloudy**?	It's cloudy, almost milky.	
	20	**Vaginal discharge?**	No.	
	21	**Back pain?**	No.	
Social Hx	22	Do you **smoke**?	No.	
(FED TACOS)	23	Do you drink **alcohol**?	No.	
	24	Do you drink **caffeine**?	I like my coffee.	
	25	How much do you drink a day?	About a pot a day.	
	26	What is your **occupation**?	I'm an author.	
	27	Are you **sexually active**?	No.	
Medical Hx	28	Do you have any medical conditions?	I have high blood pressure.	
Allergies	29	Do you have any allergies?	No.	
Surg Hx	30	Have you had any surgeries?	No.	
Hosp Hx	31	Have you ever been hospitalized?	No.	
Family Hx	32	Medical conditions that run in the family?	A little blood pressure and sugar.	
Medications	33	Are you on any medications?	Hydrochlorothiazide.	
	34	How often do you take it?	One in the morning and one at night.	
	35	How many milligrams is it?	50 mg.	

Physical Examination ✓

	36	Informs patient that the physical exam is to begin and asks permission.	
	37	Rewashes hands before touching patient if candidate has recontaminated them.	
Cardiac	38	Auscultation performed on bare skin	**Regular rhythm w/o murmur, rub, gallop**
	39	Areas: aortic, pulmonic, tricuspid, and mitral	
Respiratory	40	Auscultation performed on bare skin	**Clear to auscultation**
	41	Through complete inspiration and expiration	
	42	Symmetrically	
	43	At least 2 anterior levels, 1 lateral, and 3 posterior	
Abdominal	44	Helps patient to supine position.	
	45	Drapes lower extremities with sheet.	
	46	Inspection: Properly exposes the abdomen	**Flat**
	47	Auscultation prior to palpation	**Normoactive bowel sounds**
	48	Percussion: Four quadrants	**Tympany greatest in the LUQ**
	49	Palpation watching facial expression	**Mild tenderness in suprapubic area**
	50	CVA tenderness	**Negative**
	51	Helps patient back to seated position.	
Assessment	52	Presents patient with a proposed diagnosis.	**Urinary tract infection**
Plan	53	MTHR: Change HCTZ, antibiotic, labs with urinalysis, caffeine reduction, fluids	
(MOTHRR)	54	Return plan: Devises and explains a follow-up plan with the patient.	
	55	Thanks the patient and asks if there are any questions.	

Humanistic Evaluation   Y/N

Did the candidate present in a self-caring manner (e.g., hair control, clothing, cleanliness, aroma, etc.)?	
Did the candidate make periodic eye contact?	
Was the candidate's language clear and EASY to understand?	
Did the candidate have any substance in his or her mouth during the session?	
Did the candidate exhibit body language that would make you feel the candidate was communicating with you?	
Was the candidate enthusiastic?	
Did the candidate exhibit pride in his or her efforts?	
Did the candidate make any comment regarding your lifestyle (e.g., your work, family, activities, etc.)?	
Did the candidate express any humanistic statement recognizing your concerns?	
Did the candidate explain the medical problem and offer you a possible diagnosis?	
Did the candidate suggest a treatment plan that you could understand?	
Did the candidate inquire whether you might want to consult with family members or others about your visit?	
Did the candidate present as if he or she were a competent interviewer?	
Did the candidate ask you if you had any questions?	
Did the candidate thank you?	

COMLEX 2-PE Quick Reference Guide

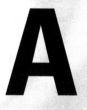
Start of 14-minute session announced	Targeted completion time (TCT) < 1 minute

Open wall unit and review:

    Patient Data Sheet: Circle abnormal BP, pulse, and respirations to be repeated during exam

    Ancillary provided data: EKGs, laboratory results, etc.

Write mnemonics on patient data sheet or provided scrap paper

    CODIERS SMASH FM

    FED TACOS

    MOTHRR

Enter the room	TCT < 1 minute

Stop a few feet inside the door, facing the patient

    Ask the patient how he or she prefers to be addressed

    Maintain eye contact

    Introduce yourself by name and title

Excuse yourself to wash your hands while explaining need to wash before touching the patient

Perform full 15-second hand washing

    Bond with patient with nonmedical conversation during hand washing

    Turn off the water with a paper towel

Return to patient

    Reintroduce yourself while shaking the patient's hand

    Sit on the examination stool, approximately 4 feet in front of the patient.

History	TCT ~ 5 minutes

Ask **"What brings you in today?"**

    Allow the story to develop and follow historical clues

    Use open-ended questions

    Maintain eye contact 50% of the time

    Follow patient comments with humanistic statements about the patient's work, family, job, ADLs

Fill in the spaces next to the associated letter in the mnemonic as history is obtained

Keep a running list of possible diagnoses as they enter the differential

Continued

Ask symptoms associated to rule in or out each possible diagnosis

When you believe the history is complete

Summarize the story with the patient

Return to blanks in the mnemonic to obtain skipped information

---

Physical Exam   TCT < 5 minutes

Ask the patient permission to start the examination

Rewash your hands if you recontaminated them

Cover the patient's lower extremities with the sheet provided if appropriate

Begin the problem-specific examination in a head-to-toe approach

Ask if each area encountered would be affected with the suspected diagnosis

Skip those areas not affected

Identify the primary absolute organ system affected

Examine in detail: inspection, auscultation, palpation, percussion

Perform examination of adjacent areas with detail as needed

Perform limited examination of distant systems of possible involvement

Advise patient of any prohibited examinations (i.e., breast, rectal, or genital) and explain that they would be recommended

2-minute warning: If you have not finished the exam, stop and proceed with the assessment

---

Assessment: Provide the patient with the proposed diagnosis.   TCT < 1 minute

---

Plan: Utilize MOTHRR mnemonic. Consider each component.   TCT ~ 2 minutes without OMM

Medications: Instruct patient on type of medication and how to take it

OMM: If appropriate, offer OMM and perform without HVLA and limited to 3 to 5 minutes

Testing: Advise patient of labs, imaging, or other testing being ordered

Holistic/Humanistic

Advise patient of RICE, work restrictions, diet changes, smoking cessation, etc.

Express concern over the condition. **Offer to involve family members**

Referrals: Advise patient if referrals are being made

Return: Advise patient of need for admission, or develop a finite follow-up plan

---

Ask the patient if he or she has any questions

Thank the patient, shaking hands

Exit the room

SOAP note documentation: 9-minute session

Begin the SOAP note immediately upon exiting the room

Do NOT document any history or examination that should have been completed but that was not. Identify them in the plan as below.

Document:

Date and time

Chief Complaint

S: Demographics

CODIERS: Paragraph form

SMASH FM: Bulleted

O: Transfer vitals from patient data sheet

Document "repeated" vitals

Systems by bulleted headings

A: **Minimum of four diagnoses related to the chief complaint in order of likelihood**

Notate less likely diagnoses by "rule out" or "doubt"

Secondary diagnoses last

P: MOTHRR format

Meds: Minimally name the class. Provide name, dose, frequency, and instructions if possible

OMM: Techniques used

Testing: Imagining, laboratory, or other testing

Referrals

Return plan

Note any history, examination, or manipulation that should have been taken or performed, but that was not done during the patient encounter.

Legible signature

Print name if not legible

If the end of session is announced at any time before you are finished, IMMEDIATELY stop and put your pencil down.

Common Medical Abbreviations

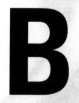
AAA	Abdominal aortic aneurysm
A&O × 3	Alert and oriented to person, place, and time
Abd	Abdomen
LLQ	Left lower quadrant
LUQ	Left upper quadrant
RLQ	Right lower quadrant
RUQ	Right upper quadrant
AD	Auric dexter (right ear)
ADLs	Activities of daily living
AKA	Also known as
AKA	Above the knee amputation
AMI	Acute myocardial infarction
AP/lat	Anteroposterior and lateral views
APAP	Acetaminophen
AROM	Active range of motion
AS	Auric sinister (left ear)
ASA	Aspirin
AU	Both ears
Bid	Twice a day
BKA	Below knee amputation
b/l	Bilateral
BPH	Benign prostatic hypertrophy
BRBPR	Bright red blood per rectum
BS	Breath sounds or bowel sounds
BSE	Breast self-examination
CABG	Coronary artery bypass graft (×2, ×3, ×4, depending on number of grafts)
CAD	Coronary artery disease
C&S	Culture and sensitivity
CC	Chief complaint

CHF	Congestive heart failure
CN II–XII	Cranial nerves II through XII
c/o	Complains of
COPD	Chronic obstructive pulmonary disease
CTA	Clear to auscultation
CVA	Cerebrovascular accident
CVA	Cost vertebral angle
CXR	Chest X-ray
D/C	Discharge
DC	Discontinued
DJD	Degenerative joint disease
DM	Diabetes mellitus
DNR	Do not resuscitate
DOA	Dead on arrival
DOB	Date of birth
DOE	Dyspnea on exertion
DTRs	Deep tendon reflexes
DUB	Dysfunctional uterine bleeding
DVT	Deep vein thrombosis
Dx	Diagnosis
EAC	External auditory canal
EGD	Esophagogastroduodenoscopy
ENT	Ear, nose, and throat
EOMI	Extraocular movements intact
ETOH	Ethanol
Ext	Extremity
FB	Foreign body
FDLNMP	First day of last normal menstrual period
FH (FHx)	Family history
FROM	Full range of motion
F/U	Follow-up
FUO	Fever of unknown origin
GI	Gastrointestinal
GU	Genitourinary
GYN	Gynecology
H/A	Headache
H&P	History and physical
HBP	High blood pressure
HEENT	Head, eyes, ears, nose, and throat
HJR	Hepatojugular reflux
H/O	History of
HPI	History of present illness
HS	At night, bedtime
HSM	Hepatosplenomegaly
HTN	Hypertension

Hx	History
I&D	Incision and drainage
IDDM	Insulin-dependent diabetes mellitus
	(also called type 1 or juvenile diabetes mellitus)
Infx	Infection
JVD	Jugular venous distention
L	Left
LLE	Left lower extremity
LLL	Left lower lobe (of lung)
LMP	Last menstrual period
LOC	Loss of consciousness
LUE	Left upper extremity
LUL	Left upper lobe (of lung)
MCL	Midclavicular line
MGF	Maternal grandfather
MGM	Maternal grandmother
MI	Myocardial infarction
m/r/g	Murmur, rub, gallop
MVA	Motor vehicle accident
NAD	No acute distress
NCAT	Normocephalic, atraumatic
NG	Nasogastric
NIDDM	Non-insulin-dependent diabetes mellitus
	(also called type 2 or adult onset diabetes mellitus)
NKA	No known allergies
NKDA	No known drug allergies
NSR	Normal sinus rhythm
N/V	Nausea and vomiting
OD	Oculus dexter (right eye)
OM	Otitis media
OS	Oculus sinister (left eye)
OTC	Over-the-counter (medication)
OU	Oculi unitas (both eyes)
PERRLA	Pupils equal, round, and reactive to light and accommodation
PGF	Paternal grandfather
PGM	Paternal grandmother
PND	Paroxysmal nocturnal dyspnea
PRN	As needed
PROM	Passive range of motion
Q	Every
QD	Every day
	(for medical legal reasons, write out, "daily" instead)
QH	Every hour

QID	Four times a day
	(for medical legal reasons, write out, "four times a day" instead)
QOD	Every other day
	(for medical legal reasons, write out, "every other day" instead)
R	Right
RA	Rheumatoid arthritis
RA	Room air
RLE	Right lower extremity
RLL	Right lower lobe (of lung)
RML	Right middle lobe (of lung)
R/O	Rule out
ROS	Review of systems
RUE	Right upper extremity
RUL	Right upper lobe (of lung)
RRR	Regular rate and rhythm
Rx	Prescription
Rxn	Reaction
SH, Soc Hx	Social history
SLR	Straight leg raising
SOAP note	Subjective, objective, assessment, and plan
SOB	Short of breath
s/p	Status post
subQ	Subcutaneously
Sx	Symptom
TID	Three times a day
TMs	Tympanic membranes
TMJ	Temporomandibular joint
TPR	Temperature, pulse, and respirations
Tx	Treatment
U/A	Urinalysis
UGI	Upper gastrointestinal
URI	Upper respiratory infection
US	Ultrasound
UTI	Urinary tract infection
VS	Vital signs
WNL	Within normal limits
WNWD	Well-nourished, well-developed

Index

A

abbreviations
  common medical, 277
  nonstandard, 55
  in SOAP notes, 55
ABCs song, during handwashing, 17
abd. *See* abdomen
abdomen (abd), 277
  examination of, 39–40, 44
abdominal pain, 27, 33, 93–96,
    241–244
  humanistic evaluation of, 96,
    204, 244
  medical history of, 203, 243
  physical examination of, 96,
    204, 244
  vital signs with, 93, 201, 241
Ache, Billy, 241
ACLS. *See* advanced cardiac life
    support
activities of daily living, 61
acute coronary syndrome, 25
admission ticket, 15
advanced cardiac life support
    (ACLS), guidelines, 14
age, of standardized patient, 15
alcohol, habits, 31
allergies, 23, 175
  medical history of, 32
  questions about, 24, 32
ambulance patient
  humanistic evaluation of, 116
  medical history of, 115
  physical examination of, 116
  vital signs of, 113
Amedus, Edward, 121
Americans with Disabilities Act, 1–2

anaphylactic reaction, 32
anatomy-based questioning, 27–28
antacid, 26
anticipated case development, 67
appearance, 11
arm pain, 229–232, 245–248
  humanistic evaluation of, 232,
    248
  medical history of, 231, 235, 247
  physical examination of, 232, 248
  vital signs with, 229, 245
assessment
  CODIERS SMASH FM in, 49
  components of, 47
  discussion of, 49
  domain of, 3
  global patient, 5
  of runny nose, 73
  scoring of, 60
  in SOAP notes, 59–60
  writing up, 55
auscultation
  for cardiac examination, 44
  CTA, 278
  of lungs, with cough, 41–42
  of respiratory system, 38, 43–44

B

back, hump on, case study of, 173
back pain, 101–105, 233–236
  humanistic evaluation of,
    104, 236
  medical history of, 103, 235
  physical examination of,
    104, 236
  vital signs with, 101
Barr, Elizabeth, 169

Bebe, Letzhavia, 125
bid. *See* twice a day
biliary system, 28
biomechanical domain, 2–3
  focus of, 13
biomedical domain, 2–3
  focus of, 13
blood pressure
  humanistic evaluation of, 132
  medical history and, 131
  physical examination of, 132
  technique for, 42
  vital signs for, 129
breast exams, 45
Brethin, Harley, 197
Bretten, Barry, 161
bronchophony, 39
Bulletin of Information, 4, 62
  summary of, 66
Bull's eye, 41
burn, on forehead, 105–108

C

caffeine, habits, 31
Candidate Confidentiality
    Agreement, 67
cardiac examination
  auscultation for, 44
  inspection for, 44
  palpation for, 39
carotids, exam of, 43
Cartia, Jack E., 257
case development
  anticipated, 67
  breakdown of, 65–67
  question development for, 65
  utilization of, 66–67

case scenario, for physical exam, 37

CC. *See* chief complaint

Chapman points, 44

chest pain, 89–93, 189–192
  humanistic evaluation of, 92, 192
  medical history of, 91, 191
  physical exam of, 92, 192
  vital signs of, 89

chief complaint (CC)
  diagnoses related to, 3
  documentation of, 57
  in history taking, 21
  occupation related to, 30
  primary diagnoses and, 47–48
  secondary diagnosis and, 48–49
  in SOAP notes, 57

Chimney, Ika, 253

cholesterol
  humanistic evaluation of, 224
  medical history of, 223
  physical examination of, 224
  vital signs with, 221

chronic obstructive pulmonary disease (COPD), 27

chronology, 23, 175
  question guide for, 23–25
  time sequencing in, 24

clear to auscultation (CTA), 278

clinical presentations, areas of, 65

clinical skills, quick review of, 273–275

CODIERS
  components of, 22–23
  documentation of, 57

CODIERS SMASH FM, 16, 22, 273
  in assessment, 49
  components of, 23

cold, common, 177
  medical history of, 111, 179
  physical examination, 112
  vital signs with, 109

COMLEX-USA Level 1
    Performance Examination, 1

COMLEX-USA Level 2 Cognitive
    Evaluation, 1

COMLEX-USA Level 2
    Performance Examination
  confidentiality agreement for, 2
  educational skills for, 7–8
  eligibility for, 1
    checklist for, 2
  expectations of, 65
  grading of, 3–4
  instructional skills for, 7–8
  listening skills for, 6–7
  resources for, 4
  respect on, 8–9

special accommodations for, 1–2
structure of, 2
testing sites for, 2
verbal skills for, 5–6

communication skills, 3

compassion, 10

confidentiality agreement
  assuring patient of, 12
  Candidate Confidentiality
    Agreement, 67
  for COMLEX exam, 2

COPD. *See* chronic obstructive pulmonary disease

cough
  auscultation for, 41–42
  humanistic evaluation of, 144, 200, 264
  medical history of, 143, 199, 263
  physical examination of, 144, 200, 264
  vitals signs with, 141, 197, 261

counterstrain, 51

cranial osteopathy, 51

CTA. *See* clear to auscultation

cyanosis, 40

D

data gathering, definition of, 13

data sheet
  patient, 14
    components of, 35–36
    example of, 16
  review of, 66

diagnosis
  -based questioning, 27
  candidate proposal of, 7–8
  CC related to, 3
  confidence in, 12
  confirmation of, tests for, 52
  primary, 47–48
  secondary, 48–49, 60
  sharing of, with patient, 49
  treatment plan after, 49–53

Dimension I Blueprint, 65

discharge, vaginal, 31

dizziness, 26

documentation
  of CC, 57
  of CODIERS, 57
  completed SOAP note example, 63
  definition of, 13
  domain of, 3
  false, 62
  of follow-up, 62
  of hospitalization, 58
  of medications, 61
  of MOTHRR, 61
  of OMM, 61

of physical examination, 59
of preexisting medical history, 60
of referrals, 62
of secondary diagnosis, 60
of SMASH FM, 58
of standardized patient, 55
of testing, 61

dosing, frequency of, 34

doubt, 60

drainage
  I&D, 279
  of sinuses, 51

dress, professional, 11

drugs, 31; *See also* medications
  questions about, 30

Dubb, Stephanie, 177

duration, of symptoms, 25–26

E

ears, exam of, 42

edema, 40
  of wrist, 165–168

educational skills, for exam, 7–8

egophony, 39

Elbel, Eddie, 229

emergency room, as office setting, 14–15

empathy
  content breakdown for, 10
  synonyms for, 10

English language, 55

epinephrine auto injector (EpiPen), 32

EpiPen. *See* epinephrine auto injector

Esper, Torrie, 97

ethics, 12

every other day (qod), 280

exacerbating factors, 23, 175
  questions about, 26

exercise, habits, 29, 31

ext. *See* extremities

extra-ocular movements fields, 43

extremities (ext)
  elapsed time examining, 40
  examination of, 40

eye contact, 10

F

facilitated positional release, 51

false documentation, 62

family history, 23, 175
  questions about, 33

family practice office, 117

fatigue
  humanistic evaluation of, 252
  medical history of, 251
  physical examination of, 252
  vital signs with, 249

fb. *See* foreign body
FDLMP. *See* first day of last
  menstrual period
FED TACOS, 29, 175, 273
  social history note taking, 30, 31
fertility planning
  humanistic evaluation for, 128
  medical history for, 127
  physical examination for, 128
  vital signs for, 125
final preparation, for patient
  encounter, 15–16
first day of last menstrual period
  (FDLMP), 32
first ring, 41
Flemming, Lucy, 141
follow-up plan, 52
  documentation of, 62
food habits, 29, 31
foot pain, 85–89, 209–212
  humanistic evaluation of, 88, 212
  medical history of, 87, 211
  physical examination of, 88, 212
  vital signs with, 85, 209
forehead burn, 105–108
  humanistic evaluation of, 108
  medical history of, 107
  physical examination of, 108
  vital signs with, 105
foreign body (fb), 278
forgetfulness
  humanistic evaluation of, 84
  medical history of, 83
  physical examination of, 84
  vital signs with, 81
four times a day (qid), 280
Freqaunty, Mary Jo, 269
frequency
  of dosing, 34
  of urination, 269–272
Furtz, Cal, 205

G
Gaine, Tom, 213
galbreath technique, 51
gallbladder, questions about,
  27–28
genital exams, 45
global patient assessment, 5
grading, of exam, 3–4
Grates, Farah, 109
grooming, 11

H
handwashing
  length of, 17–18
  technique for, 17
happy birthday song, during
  handwashing, 17
Hart, Tracy, 225

headache
  humanistic evaluation of, 148,
    151, 268
  medical history of, 147, 151, 267
  physical examination of, 148,
    151, 268
  vital signs with, 145, 149, 265
head-to-toe method, of physical
  exam, 37–40
health maintenance, issue with, 60
hearing loss
  humanistic evaluation of, 216
  medical history of, 215
  physical examination of, 216
  vital signs with, 213
hearing tests, 43
heart
  beat, irregular, 257–260
  elapsed time examining, 40
  failure of
    medications treating, 27
    physical exam for, 38
HEENT exam, 42
hematuria
  humanistic evaluation of, 220
  medical history of, 219
  physical examination of, 220
  vital signs with, 217
hepatojugular reflex, 40
Hertz, Harmon, 75
history (Hx), 279; *See also* medical
  history
*History and Physical
  Examination: A Common
  Sense Approach*, 55
history of present illness (HPI), 19
  components of, 22–34
  prior, 24
history taking
  CC in, 21
  domain of, 3
  logical sequence in, 21–22
  question asking in, 19
  redirection in, 20
Ho, Mau, 261
holistic treatment, 52
  in SOAP notes, 61
hospitalization, 23, 175
  documentation of, 58
  history of, 33
HPI. *See* history of present illness
humanistic domain, 3
  focus of, 5
  in SOAP notes, 61
humanistic evaluation, 176, 180,
    184, 188
  of abdominal pain, 96, 204, 244
  of ambulance patient, 116
  of arm pain, 232, 248
  of back pain, 104, 236

of blood pressure, 132
of chest pain, 92, 192
of cholesterol, 224
of cold, 112
of cough, 144, 200, 264
of fatigue, 252
of fertility planning, 128
of foot pain, 88, 212
of forehead burn, 108
of forgetfulness, 84
of headache, 148, 151, 268
of hearing loss, 216
of hematuria, 220
of irregular heart beat, 260
of knee pain, 140
of leg pain, 124, 208
of lightheadedness, 160
of neck pain, 156
of palpitations, 228
of pregnancy, 240
of rash, 172
of runny nose, 72
of shortness of breath, 100, 164
of shoulder pain, 78
of smoking, 256
of spitting up, 136
of urinary tract infection, 120
of wrist swelling, 168
humanistic treatment, 52, 61
HVLA techniques, 51
Hx. *See* history

I
I&D. *See* incision and drainage
incision and drainage (I&D), 279
infection (Infx), 279
Infx. *See* infection
instructional skills, for exam, 7–8
integumentary system,
  examination of, 42
intensity, 23
  of symptoms, 26
interpersonal skills, 3
introduction to, 16–17
Iskus, Emmanuel, 137

J
*Journal of American Osteopathic
  Association*, 67

K
Karfle, Betty B., 145
knee pain, 137–140
  humanistic evaluation of, 140
  medical history of, 139
  physical examination of, 140
  vital signs with, 137
knee trauma, 35
Kno, Ida, 81
Koppe, Sid, 157

L

language, English, 55
Laturel, Junie, 149
leg pain, 121–124, 205–208
  humanistic evaluation of, 124,
    208
  lower, 181
    medical history of, 183
  medical history of, 123, 207
  physical examination of, 124,
    208
  vital signs with, 121, 205
lightheadedness
  humanistic evaluation of, 160
  medical history of, 159
  physical examination of, 160
  vital signs of, 157
listening skills, breakdown of, 6–7
Little, Eileen A., 113
liver, questions about, 28
logical sequence, in history taking,
  21–22
lungs
  auscultation of, with cough,
    41–42
  elapsed time examining, 40
  examination of, 39
  tumor of, 60
lymphatic techniques, 51

M

medical abbreviations, common,
  277
medical history, 22–23
  of abdominal pain, 203, 243
  of allergies, 32
  of ambulance patient, 115
  of arm pain, 231, 235, 247
  of back pain, 103, 235
  of blood pressure, 131
  of chest pain, 91, 191
  of cholesterol, 223
  of common cold, 111, 179
  of cough, 143, 199, 263
  of fatigue, 251
  of fertility, 127
  of foot pain, 87, 211
  of forehead burn, 107
  of forgetfulness, 83
  of headache, 147, 151, 267
  of hearing loss, 215
  of hematuria, 219
  of knee pain, 137–140
  of leg pain, 123, 207
  of lightheadedness, 159
  of lower leg pain, 183
  of neck pain, 155
  of palpitations, 227
  preexisting, 60
  of pregnancy, 239

  of private problem, 195
  questions about, 32
  of rash, 171
  of runny nose, 71
  of shortness of breath, 99, 163
  of shoulder pain, 77
  of smoking, 255
  of spitting up, 135
  of urinary tract infection, 119
  of urination, 270
  of wrist swelling, 167
medical school, osteopathic, 1
medications, 23, 175; *See also*
  drugs
  documentation of, 61
  problems from, 50
  questions about, 33–34
  in SOAP notes, 61
  treating heart failure, 27
  in treatment plan, 49–50
Mei, Carrie, 181
Mencies, Melissa, 185
menses, lack of, 185
MOTHRR, 273–274
  components of, 49–53
  documentation of, 61
  in SOAP notes, 61
Moto, Kali, 173
Motrin, 50
mouth, exam of, 43
muscle(s)
  energy techniques, 51
  strength of, testing of, 44
musculoskeletal examination, 40
  osteopathic, 44
myofascial techniques, 51

N

name of, 14
nasal congestion, 57
National Board of Osteopathic
  Medical Examiners (NBOME),
  1, 65
NBOME. *See* National Board of
  Osteopathic Medical
  Examiners
neck, examination of, 38, 40, 43
neck pain
  humanistic evaluation of, 156
  medical history of, 155
  physical examination of, 156
  vital signs with, 153
neurologic examination, 40, 44–45
nonstandard abbreviations, 55
nose, runny, 26, 69–73

O

obstetric history, 187
occupation, 29, 31
  CC related to, 30

office setting
  emergency room as, 14–15
  practice cases simulated in, 66
office visit, reason for, 15
OM. *See* osteopathic manipulation
OMM. *See* osteopathic
  manipulative medicine
OMT. *See* osteopathic
  manipulative treatment
onset, 23, 175
  changes since, 24
  question guide for, 23–25
O'Pen, Terry, 189
open-ended questions
  introduction to, 19
  use of, 20
opening statement, 19
ophthalmoscopic exam, 43
osteopathic manipulation (OM), 50
osteopathic manipulative medicine
  (OMM), 2
  documentation of, 61
  domain of, 3
  indications for, 50
  scoring for, 51
  techniques used for, 50–51
osteopathic manipulative
  treatment (OMT)
  definition of, 13
  guidelines for, 51
  recommended techniques
    for, 51
osteopathic medical school, 1
  NBOME, 1
osteopathic musculoskeletal
  examination, 44
otitis externa, 31
otoscopic exam, 42

P

pain
  abdominal, 27, 33, 93–96,
    241–244
  case study of, 201–204
  in arm, 229–232, 245–248
  in back, 101–105, 233–236
  in chest, 89–93, 189–192
  in foot, 85–89, 209–212
  in knee, 137–140
  in leg, 121–124, 205–208
  lower leg, 181, 183
  in neck, 153, 155–156
  in shoulder, 75–79
Paine, Chester, 89
palpation, 38
  for cardiac evaluation, 39
  for respiratory evaluation, 39
palpitations
  humanistic evaluation of, 228
  medical history of, 227

physical examination of, 228
vitals signs with, 225
Pean, Barry, 193
pectoriloquy, 39
penicillin, 32
percussion, for respiratory system, 39, 44
Pfodz, Patricia, 221
physical appearance, 11
physical examination; *See also specific examination i.e. vascular examination*
of abdominal pain, 96, 204, 244
of ambulance patient, 116
of arm pain, 232, 248
of back pain, 104, 236
of blood pressure, 132
case scenario for, 37
of chest pain, 92, 192
for cholesterol, 224
of cold, 112
of cough, 144, 200, 264
documentation of, 59
domain of, 3
elapsed time for, sample of, 40
of fatigue, 252
for fertility planning, 128
of foot pain, 88, 212
of forehead burn, 108
of forgetfulness, 84
of headache, 148, 151, 268
head-to-toe method of, 37–40
of hearing loss, 216
for heart failure, 38
of hematuria, 220
of irregular heart beat, 260
of knee pain, 140
of leg pain, 124, 208
of lightheadedness, 160
methods of, 37
of neck pain, 156
of palpitations, 228
in practice case, 68
of pregnant patient, 240
problem specific, 35
prohibited, 41
proper, 59
questions before starting, 36–37
quick review of, 274
of rash, 172
relevant, 39
for runny nose, 72
of sensitive areas, 45
for shoulder pain, 78
of smoking, 256
in SOAP notes, 59
of sob, 100, 164
of spitting up, 136
of standardized patient, 35
target method of, 40–41

techniques of, 38
tips for, by system, 41–45
of urinary tract infection, 120
of wrist swelling, 168
physician position, 51
plan; *See also* fertility planning
domain of, 3
follow-up, 52
of treatment, 31
after diagnosis, 49–53
exit after, 53
pneumonia, 28
practice case
physical exams in, 68
SOAP notes in, 67
summary of, 67
Prayn, Frank, 233
pregnancy
humanistic evaluation of, 240
medical history of, 239
physical exam of, 240
vital signs with, 237
primary diagnoses, CC and, 47–48
private problem, 193
medical history for, 195
professional dress, 11
professionalism, 3
content breakdown for, 11–12
standardized patient checklist for, 11
prohibited physical examination, 41
pseudomonas, 31
pupillary reaction, tests for, 43

Q

qid. *See* four times a day
qod. *See* every other day
questions
about allergies, 24, 32
anatomy-based, 27–28
development, for case development, 65
diagnosis-based, 27
about drugs, 30
exacerbating factors about, 26
about family history, 33
about gallbladder, 27–28
in history taking, 19
about liver, 28
about medical history, 32
about medications, 33–34
about onset, 23–25
open-ended, 19–20
remitting factors about, 26
sequencing of, 22
shingles associated, 27
for starting physical examination, 36–37
about surgical history, 32–33

thought process behind, 22
time sequencing of, 24
about ulceration, 28

R

rash
humanistic evaluation of, 172
medical history of, 171
physical examination of, 172
vital signs with, 169
rectal exams, 45
redirection, in history taking, 20
referrals, 52
documentation of, 62
reflexes
examination of, 45
viscerosomatic, 44
remission, 175
remitting factors, 23
about questions, 26
respect
breakdown of, 8–9
definition of, 8–9
for standardized patient, 9–10
standardized patient checklist for, 9
respiratory system
inspection/auscultation of, 38, 43–44
palpation for, 39
percussion for, 39, 44
rest, ice, compression, and elevation (RICE), 52
return visit, 52
review of systems (ROS), 26–27
problem-specific, 29
Rhinne test, 43
RICE. *See* rest, ice, compression, and elevation
Rieno, Rita, 69
right to choose, 9
risk factor, 60
ROS. *See* review of systems
Rule out, 60
runny nose, 26
assessment of, 73
humanistic evaluation of, 72
medical history of, 71
physical examination for, 72
SOAP notes for, 73
vital signs with, 69

S

scoring
of assessment, 60
for OMM, 51
of SOAP notes, 64
second ring, 41
secondary diagnosis, 48–49
documentation of, 60

sensitive exams, 45
sensory examination, 44
sex, of standardized patient, 15
sexual history, 31, 187
    FDLMP in, 32
shingles, questions associated
    with, 27
shortness of breath (sob)
    humanistic evaluation of, 100,
      164
    medical history of, 99, 163
    physical examination of, 100, 164
    vital signs with, 97, 161
shoulder pain, 75–79
    humanistic evaluation of, 78
    medical history for, 77
    physical examination for, 78
    SOAP notes for, 79
    vital signs with, 75
sinus drainage techniques, 51
SMASH FM, 22
    components of, 29–30
    documentation of, 58
    in SOAP notes, 58
smoking
    humanistic evaluation of, 256
    medical history of, 255
    physical examination of, 256
    vital signs with, 253
SOAP notes. See subjective,
    objective, assessment, plan
sob. See shortness of breath
social history, 23, 29–30, 175, 187
    note taking: FED TACOS, 30, 31
somatic dysfunction, 44, 60
Soore, Nneka, 153
Spectin, Ima, 237
Spencer technique, 51
spitting up
    humanistic evaluation of, 136
    medical history of, 135
    physical examination of, 136
    vital signs with, 133
standardized patient
    age of, 15
    background of, 9
    documentation of, 55
    empathy for, 10
    encounters with
      final preparation for, 15–16
      overview of, 13–14
    physical examination of, 35
    professionalism checklist for, 11
    prohibited physical examination
      on, 41
    respect for, 9–10
    right to choose, 9
    sex of, 15
    verbal skills checklist of, 6
    video recordings of, 62

vital signs of, 15, 36
still technique, 51
Stoner, Gail, 201
subjective, objective, assessment,
    plan (SOAP notes)
    abbreviations in, 55
    assessment in, 59–60
    blank, example of, 56
    CC in, 57
    CODIERS in, 57
    completed, sample of, 63
    completion time for, 55
    components of, 57
    date on, 55
    on exam, 2
    factual information on, 59
    holistic/humanistic care in, 61
    incomplete, 64
    medications in, 61
    mistakes on, 58
    MOTHRR in, 61
    negative findings in, 59
    objective in, 58–59
    physical examination in, 59
    positive findings in, 58
    in practice cases, 67
    quick review of, 274
    for runny nose, 73
    scoring of, 64
    for shoulder pain, 79
    SMASH FM in, 58
    start of, 13–14
    subjective in, 19, 55
    testing in, 61
    time allowed for, 62
    writing, 55
Sun, Theodora, 265
surgical history, 23, 175
    questions about, 32–33
swelling, 40
    of wrist, 165–168
sympathy, 10
symptoms, 175
    associated, 23, 26–27
      with specific systems, 29
    description of, 25–26
    duration of, 25–26
    intensity of, 26
    order of, 24

T
target completion time, quick
    review of, 273–275
target method, of physical exam,
    40–41
Tentson, Hiram, 129
testing
    for diagnosis confirmation, 52
    documentation of, 61
    of hearing, 43

of muscles, 44
    for pupillary reaction, 43
    Rhinne, 43
    sites for, 2
    in SOAP notes, 61
    for visual acuity, 43
thrust techniques, 51
thyroid, exam of, 43
Tinter, Ness, 85
tissue texture changes, 44
tobacco, habits, 31
Todd, Ruby, 165
Torres, Sakrel, 101
Train, Fred, 249
trauma, to knee, 35
treatment
    holistic/humanistic, 52, 61
    length of, 51
    OMT, 13, 51
    plan of, 31
      after diagnosis, 49–53
      exit after, 53
    timing of, 52
Trippen, Emma, 245
tumor, lung, 60
twice a day (bid), 277

U
ulceration, questions about, 28
Ulrich, Crystal, 209
urgent care, 209
urinary tract infection (uti)
    humanistic evaluation of, 120
    medical history of, 119
    physical examination of, 120
    vital signs with, 117
urination
    frequency of, 269–272
    medical history of, 270
    problems with, 195–196
Urn, Buddy, 217
uti. See urinary tract infection

V
vaginal discharge, 31
vascular examination, 44
verbal skills
    breakdown of, 5–6
    standardized patient checklist
      for, 6
video recordings, of standardized
    patient, 62
viscerosomatic reflexes, 44
visual acuity, tests for, 43
vital signs
    with abdominal pain, 93, 201,
      241
    of ambulance patient, 113
    with arm pain, 229, 245
    with back pain, 101

with blood pressure, 129
with chest pain, 89
with cholesterol, 221
with common cold, 109
with cough, 141, 197, 261
elapsed time examining, 40
with fatigue, 249
for fertility planning, 125
with foot pain, 85, 209
with forehead burn, 105
with forgetfulness, 81
with headache, 145, 149, 265
with hearing loss, 213
with hematuria, 217
with knee pain, 137
with leg pain, 121, 205

with lightheadedness, 157
with neck pain, 153
normal ranges for, 36
with palpitations, 225
with pregnancy, 237
with rash, 169
review of, 36
with runny nose, 69
with shortness of breath, 97, 161
with shoulder pain, 75
with smoking, 253
with spitting up, 133
of standardized patient, 15, 36
technique for, 42
with urinary tract infection, 117
with wrist swelling, 165

W
wall unit, 15
    review of, 1
Wilhapen, Ester, 105
wrist swelling, 165–168
    humanistic evaluation of, 168
    medical history of, 167
    physical examination of, 168
    vital signs with, 165

Y
Yoria, Polly, 117
Yupp, Chuckie, 133

Z
Zahurtin, Jim, 93